W9-BVO-450

THE NEWMAN'S OWN ORGANICS GUIDE TO A GOOD LIFE

THE
NEWMAN'S OWN®
ORGANICS
GUIDE
TO A
GOOD LIFE

Simple Measures
That Benefit You
and the Place You Live

Nell Newman

with Joseph D'Agnese

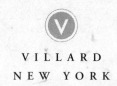

VILLARD

NEW YORK

All rights reserved under International and Pan-American Copyright Conventions.
Published in the United States by Villard Books, a division of Random House, Inc.,
New York, and simultaneously in Canada by
Random House of Canada Limited, Toronto.

VILLARD and CIRCLED "V" Design are
registered trademarks of Random House, Inc.

Library of Congress Cataloging-in-Publication Data

Newman, Nell.
The Newman's Own Organics guide to a good life: simple measures that benefit you
and the place you live / Nell Newman with Joseph D'Agnese.
p.   cm.
Includes bibliographical references and index.
ISBN 0-8129-6733-X
1. Organic living. 2. Human ecology. 3. Environmental protection. 4. Conservation of
natural resources. I. D'Agnese, Joseph. II. Newman's Own Organics. III. Title.
GF77 .N49 2003   640—dc21   2002033128

Villard website address: www.villard.com

Printed in the United States of America on New Leaf Eco Book 100,
which is made with 100% postconsumer recycled fibers and processed chlorine free

24689753

FIRST EDITION

Book design by Carole Lowenstein

For my mother and father

Acknowledgments

First and foremost, I want to thank Peter Meehan, my friend and business partner, without whom Newman's Own Organics would not exist; Sally Shepard, my press relations person extraordinaire, who coaches me patiently through my life in the public arena; and everyone in the office at Newman's Own Organics for all their valuable feedback. Thanks to Alice Waters for her inspiration and relentless encouragement from the very beginning; and Maggie Waldron, who is much missed, from Ketchum Communications, whose marketing expertise and high standards pushed us to be our best.

Enormous thanks to Joe D'Agnese, my co-author, for his tireless work, humor, intelligence, enthusiasm, and commitment to this project. You've been fantastic.

James Cox, my longtime friend, helped shape many of the ideas in this book; Bob Scowcroft, my friend and confidant in the world of organic agriculture, provided expert input; Jack Silbert assisted with occasional comedic bits; and Lori Garth offered expert assistance locating reference materials and providing input.

My appreciation to the crew at Random House—Dennis Ambrose, Carole Lowenstein, Misa Erder, Stacy Rockwood, and Alexa Cassanos—for their exceptional care throughout every

 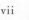

stage of publication, and to Mary Bahr, my editor, without whom this book would never have happened.

Thanks, also, to Gary Irving, whose moral support gave me much encouragement.

I don't have words enough to thank the two people to whom this book is dedicated, my mother and father, whose example taught me to care.

Contents

Contents

  x

Introduction

I never expected to write this kind of book. In fact, I seldom read this kind of book. When I thought about that apparent inconsistency, given my interest in ecology and the environment, I realized that the book I wanted to read did not exist. I think that reading a book full of "shoulds" would be almost as tedious as writing one. Yet I also believe that it's worthwhile to share stories, trade ideas, and exchange not only encouragement but also down-to-earth advice with people who care about their own well-being and the health of the planet.

With that in mind, let me confess up front that this book is not without contradictions. In fact, the printed book itself—100 percent postconsumer recycled paper and soy ink notwithstanding—is a contradiction. It took resources to produce it and get it to you. Every positive measure you take to help the environment probably entails a downside. You might order fair-trade organic cotton clothing over the Internet to support this worthy business model, but getting that item involves energy-expensive packaging and shipping. You might go out of your way to buy organic food, but driving farther means emitting more pollutants into the air and using extra fuel. It's fairly obvious that one can't be a "perfect" environmentalist. But that's okay. Perfection isn't the goal. A good life is. And a good life has a lot to do with who you are in the world, with your intent as much as with the end result.

I don't expect you to make use of every suggestion offered in these pages, nor do I intend it to be a definitive encyclopedia of living green. My aim is to inspire you as you read about people who have done some fascinating and sometimes hilarious things to live more in tune with nature. I hope that among the steps outlined at the end of each chapter you will identify those that are within reach for you. You are probably already doing some of them, and you might have suggestions for me, too. Enjoy yourself and live a little. If you slavishly reuse every paper bag that comes your way until it's a pulpy wad, go ahead and issue yourself some "environmental credits" to spend on taking a spin in your sporty guzzler.

A good life, after all, isn't one of relentless deprivation. Quite the opposite. I've discovered that caring for the world around me rewards me more than my small effort really deserves. So I hope it's not too crass to admit that my seemingly altruistic choices are not entirely so. The selfish benefits of living an environmentally conscious life are many. Through supporting organic growers by eating organic produce, I enjoy much more delicious and healthful food. When I walk rather than drive to run errands, I get exercise and sunshine (okay, I know I'm spoiled here in Santa Cruz). When I use biodegradable cleaners and detergents for my clothes and in my home, I reduce my exposure to toxic chemicals. And most of all, whatever small thing I do for someone else is often paid back many times over in humbling ways.

In the course of researching this book I discovered many things I didn't know. I came across suggestions for saving energy, water, time, money, and fuel—you name it—that were new to me. I also found myself more excited about practicing what I already know to do. As you browse these pages I hope that will be your experience too.

THE NEWMAN'S OWN ORGANICS GUIDE TO A GOOD LIFE

CHAPTER 1

FOOD

There is a communion of more than our bodies
when bread is broken and wine drunk.
—M. F. K. Fisher

I was lucky to have grown up in an old colonial farmhouse with a garden and a few apple trees. My mom taught me to cook at an early age, and the ingredients we used came from our garden. The fruit of those trees ended up in our pies, and the eggs laid by our chickens went into cakes and omelets. My father taught me to fish, and we polished off what I plucked out of the Aspetuck River with corn and tomatoes from a local farm stand. My pa always had a good eye for produce. Early on, he showed me how to thump a melon.

But he still had some stubborn views about food. To him, organic foods referred to the hippie-dippy dishes my mom experimented with in the sixties, like nut loaf with yeast gravy. He was due for a wake-up call.

As my own food awareness grew, I'd gradually begun using organic ingredients in my cooking. And for some time I had been trying to get my father to add an organics line to his food company. But whenever I brought up the subject, he dismissed it because he didn't really understand organics. I was on a mission to change his mind.

My father expected a traditional Thanksgiving meal, and I was going to give him one. Sort of. One year, before leaving California to go home to Connecticut, I packed a bunch of organic foods from my local haunts. Petite pois. Sweet potatoes. Bread crumbs for stuffing. The whole bit, down to the turkey, packed in ice. I flew home with this cornucopia in my luggage and headed straight for the kitchen.

When the meal was over and I could see that it more than met with his approval, I leaned over and asked my pa, "How did you like your organic Thanksgiving meal?" He was floored. That was the day he learned that there is nothing newfangled about organic food. If anything, it's downright old-fashioned, and its rules for coaxing food from the earth date back almost ten thousand years, to the invention of agriculture. That was perhaps the most thankful Thanksgiving my family had enjoyed together up to that time. My four sisters and my mom were in on the conspiracy and supportive of my goal. We looked at my father—content, well fed, ready to embrace the ideas of modern organics, which are instinctive and simple but require a new paradigm in order to be incorporated into our high-tech and complex food culture.

Most of the time, what we eat is removed from where and how it is produced. Convenience often takes precedence over taste, nutrition, and the consequences of production and delivery. Most of us don't know or don't think about where our food originates and are not aware that eating is, as the farmer, author, and poet Wendell Berry says, "an agricultural act."

The organic movement is gaining momentum. Today you can go to any major city in the United States and eat at top-flight restaurants where chefs use only organic meats and produce. You dine exquisitely in these places; out-of-towners book reservations months in advance. There are now two major natural-food-store chains dotting the country, and you can also order organic foodstuffs online. Americans are rediscovering their local farmers, either at regional markets or through an innovative concept called Community Supported Agriculture (CSA).

The chief difference between organic and conventional food is the method used to grow or make it. No long-lasting, synthetic pesticides or herbicides are sprayed on organic veggies and fruits. The livestock grow without hormones meant to fatten them quickly and without antibiotics to keep them from getting sick in overcrowded feedlots. The land and feed is also certified organic. On organic farms the soil, water, air, and all living creatures (including humans) are spared the stress of assimilating compounds that are proving unnecessarily complex and threatening. Biological reality has proven that volume and price are poor substitutes for a healthy ecosystem.

Few of us realize that the American way of producing food has become one of the biggest threats to the environment. The apple you buy in Maryland was picked in Washington State and flown, hauled by rail, or trucked to your store. Other foods—like canned veggies and cereals—are overprocessed, overpackaged, and overpreserved for this journey and extended shelf life. By the time you eat the typical bowl of cereal, the wheat, corn, or oats have been stripped of their nutrient value and coated with sugar and preservatives. Meanwhile, the harvesters, conveyors, packing machines, trucks, and other devices that make all this happen demand fuel, and so they too take their toll on our resources and the air we breathe. Yes, the food gets to where it has to go, but it's hardly efficient. By one estimate, for every calorie we eat, ten calories of energy have been used to bring it to us.

Modern farms grow food the way factories build widgets. Technology, not the earth's natural rhythm, is assumed to hold the answer to every problem. Want bigger yields? Use this industrial fertilizer. Want to eradicate bugs? Spray these chemicals. The irony is, after decades of these practices, the bugs are only getting stronger and the land is less fertile. In many parts of the country the soil is literally drying up and washing away.

We might wonder why any farmer would employ such self-defeating methods, but the American farmer no longer holds the keys to his or her own future. The suicide rate among farmers and ranchers is three times the national average. Shattered families and ruined soil are the unfortunate legacies of corporate agribusiness. In 1920, 80 percent of the consumer's dollar went directly to the farmer. Now it's 10 percent. Since 1969, we've lost 800,000 small farms.

WHAT THE BIRDS HAVE TAUGHT ME

It's a long way from the days my parents remember, when families ate food they grew or raised themselves, supplemented with stuff they got from local farmers or shopkeepers. Back then, the distance traveled from the land to your lips was surprisingly short, and the farmer pocketed a fair wage. Those days are largely gone, and I must have been eleven years old when I first became conscious of the shift away from this way of life. For one thing, the farm stand and orchard where we used to buy our produce was sold to developers, and the first condos came to town. Then I learned that my favorite bird—the peregrine falcon—faced extinction because of DDT, the first synthetic pesticide of the postwar era.

Starting in 1942, entire neighborhoods in the United States were sprayed with DDT, and kids thought it was fun to play in the mist coming off the big spray trucks as they trolled suburbia. What no one knew, not even the Swiss scientist who won a Nobel Prize for discovering its lethality, was that this toxin was so long-lasting that it could hitch a ride up the food chain from insect to bird to predator, or from livestock to human. In other words, the more small birds a falcon hunted and ate, the more DDT was stored in its fatty tissues. As it accumulates, DDT becomes more concentrated and causes birds to lay eggs with thinner shells in addition to adversely affecting their reproductive behavior. All over the country, mother peregrines, bald eagles, and ospreys crushed their eggs while incubating them. And several generations of these species were nearly wiped out.

When I grew up, I studied human ecology and worked to restore the peregrine falcon to its natural habitat. Eggs thinned by DDT were removed from nests and hatched in incubators, and the babies were returned to their mothers. The eggs that didn't hatch were analyzed for contaminants. The other scientists and I thought it would be interesting to test our own blood for background levels as we did with the eggs. We all tested positive for various contaminants, mine being DDT, PCBs, and chlordane. It

Meet the Dirty Dozen

Throughout this book, you'll hear me rail against chemicals that are harming our bodies, food, and environment. I would rather not make such sweeping generalizations, but since seventy to eighty thousand chemicals have been unleashed on the planet since World War II, it gets kind of tough to point to each by name. These twelve have been singled out by the United Nations Environmental Program as the most pernicious. They don't readily deteriorate, they remain in the environment decades after application, and they are absorbed by living organisms. Some on this list are banned in the United States; others, such as dioxins, are very much with us.

POLLUTANT	YEAR INTRODUCED	PRIMARY USE*
Aldrin	1949	Insecticide
Chlordane	1945	Insecticide
DDT	1942	Insecticide
Dieldrin	1948	Insecticide
Endrin	1951	Rodenticide, insecticide
Heptachlor	1948	Insecticide
Hexachlorabenzene	1945	Insecticide
Mirex	1959	Insecticide, fire retardant
Toxaphene	1948	Insecticide
PCBs	1929	Industrial chemical
Dioxin	1920s	Industrial by-product
Furans	1920s	Industrial by-product

*Some chemicals have or had multiple applications.
(Source: Worldwatch Institute, Paper 153)

didn't matter that I was only about thirty years old and eating mostly organic food. Background levels are everywhere, and chemicals are ubiquitous in all of us.

All three of these chemicals, now banned in the United States, are found on the United Nations' "dirty dozen" list of the most dangerous chemicals known to man. Banning them is a good first step, but it doesn't solve the problem. Once these chemicals are released into the atmosphere, they take decades to deteriorate, and they remain lethal the entire time.

There's a cruel metaphor at work here. As I learned when I had my blood tested, what happens to the birds happens in time to us. It's impossible to avoid these chemicals. But with us the agent of our ruin is invisible. We don't hatch our young from eggs, but DDT and other dirty chemicals are transmissible through foods, water, and even human breast milk. Many of these pesticides mimic hormones in the body.

So when people ask, "Why organic?," I explain that it's safer for you, better for the environment. We are all tied to the earth in a vast web of life, and what happens to the lowliest of creatures eventually touches us.

I offer my opinion because the definitive "smoking gun" study does not yet exist. But in 2002 a study led by *Consumer Reports* analyzed data from ninety-four thousand food samples. The findings showed that organically grown foods contain far fewer pesticide residues than those produced using "conventional" toxic pesticides, herbicides, and synthetic fertilizers.

While we can do very little about the toxins already lurking in our soil and water, we can definitely stop adding more. The most inspiring news regarding this national travesty is that thousands of small organic farmers are farming their parcels of land in a manner our grandparents and great-grandparents would easily recognize. The rest of us can support them by buying the fruits of their safe, nutritious harvests. By choosing organics and shopping at your local farmers market, you can get to know exactly who grew your food.

GMOs—My Biggest Concern

One of my biggest concerns is the unannounced, unlabeled, untested, and, until recently, largely unregulated introduction of

GMOs (genetically modified organisms) into the nation's food supply. GMOs or GE (genetically engineered) products are made when microbiologists insert the genetic material from one species into the DNA of another with the aim of introducing positive characteristics. Biotechnologists claim that this process is no different from the selective breeding of plants and animals that man has conducted for thousands of years. They argue that bioengineered food will eliminate or radically reduce the use of pesticides, that the use of these seeds will reduce the cost of farming, and that we need to develop this expertise in order to feed the world's growing population. All of these claims are unproven at best.

Many of the companies that are sponsoring, and profiting from, the use of GMOs are the very same ones that developed the pesticides and contaminants now found as background levels in our blood. It was twenty years before we realized that DDT nearly eliminated entire bird populations—the peregrine falcon, the brown pelican, and the bald eagle. It took millions of dollars, decades of monitoring, and captive breeding projects to restore these species. And we are only now beginning to understand the effects of these chemicals on our own health. Because biotechnology is a fairly new field, the ramifications of cross-species breeding are unknown. Important questions need to be addressed.

For example, corn that is bioengineered to produce its own toxin (Bt corn) kills the insects that eat it. That sounds good unless you happen to be an untargeted species such as a monarch, tiger swallowtail, or a fritillary butterfly whose larvae may consume the affected pollen. What are the long-term effects on these populations of insects? Another concern is the effects on the beneficial organisms found in soil once the roots of Bt crops decay. No one knows because the question has not been fully studied.

In addition, bioengineered foods do not preclude the use of toxic pesticides and herbicides. Monsanto is a leading global biotechnology company that produces many kinds of GMO seeds, including seeds engineered to withstand higher doses of Roundup herbicide (a weed killer). While Monsanto's Bt corn can be raised without using pesticides, many of their other agricultural crops, such as soybeans and cotton, have been bioengineered to be resistant to Roundup. This makes it possible to spray twice as often without killing the crop. Most frightening, whereas pesticides—undesirable as they are—degrade over time, bioengineered crops may perpetuate themselves. They spread their genes via pollen as far as the wind can blow or a bird can fly.

Biological concerns aside, GMOs represent yet another intrusion of corporate control into the American landscape. The biggest chemical companies in the land now own our seed companies. Planting a GM crop entails a licensing agreement with the seed company. Farmers agree to use it for one season only. If they save the best seeds to plant again—something farmers have done for thousands of years—they can be sued. So each year farmers are obliged to buy more seed, increasing their dependence on these companies.

Those who now control the seeds promise us revolutionary plants to end hunger, eradicate vitamin deficiencies, and withstand storms and droughts in developing nations. But research now shows that organic farms can match conventional ones for productivity, and outperform them during droughts. Moreover, food *distribution,* not food *production,* is the biggest obstacle to ending world hunger.

The European Union, Japan, Brazil, Hungary, and many other countries have either made the decision not to plant genetically engineered crops at all, or instituted a moratorium until further studies determine the safety and overall effects of these crops. For reasons that remain unknown to rational Americans, our government decided that the public did not need to know about this change in our food production. As people begin to find out, concern is growing. So ubiquitous are GM foods that the only way to know for certain that your food is grown and processed without the use of GM seeds is to buy certified organic food. And doing so sends a booming message to agribusiness.

Soil Man

Even if you've got the brownest thumb in the world, you do know one or two things about plants. You know they need nutrients, water, and something to keep away the bugs. Conventional agriculture purports to give plants all three of these things, but as you'll see, the methods used are not sustainable. They don't cooperate with natural processes and ultimately do more harm than good. Organic farmers, by contrast, mimic the earth's own processes for long-term health and renewal.

To be honest, it's not rocket science. Just ask Scott Chaskey. He runs Quail Hill Farm on Long Island, New York, which is a project of the Peconic Land Trust, an organization that has preserved more than five thousand total acres in Long Island. Scott's a good-natured guy who looks a little like a rail-thin Santa Claus. He is a member of a loose network of small farmers participating in Community Supported Agriculture. Through this program, every year a bunch of people get together and buy a "share" in Scott's harvest. Once the crops start coming in, they'll drop by the farm to pick up their vegetables, herbs, and fruits. Since the farm is pretty small and easily reached by members nearby, all the shareholders actually go into the fields and pick their own, but that's something of a rarity among CSAs. Other CSA farms organize drop-off points in nearby towns.

"The biggest advantage," says Scott, "is that the members are sharing the risk with the farmer. So, say one year I don't have a good garlic or potato crop, but I have a great year for carrots and greens. That's reflected in what the members eat."

Already, we can start to see the difference between Scott's farm and ones run by farmers who sell to the big food producers. Scott plants crops the way portfolio managers pick stocks: he diversifies his holdings so he's never fully invested in any one thing. He grows greens, lettuces, herbs, carrots, potatoes, garlic—pretty much everything the average American wants to have in the kitchen when making a meal. This is the way small American farms used to look and indeed how most backyard vegetable gardens still look today.

Conventional large-scale farming, on the other hand, focuses instead on growing a single crop such as corn, wheat, or soybeans. The farmers who work this way use chemical fertilizers and pesticides to get their high yields. Pesticides do not discriminate; they kill the good bugs along with the bad ones. Industrial fertilizers supply three essential nutrients to plants—nitrogen, potassium, and phosphorus—and little else. It would be like you and me swallowing multivitamins and not eating three meals a day. More fertilizer is needed the next year, and soil is depleted. U.S. farms have lost an average of 1.7 billion tons of soil every year. Over time, strong salts in the fertilizers kill the microorganisms that live in the soil. Everything in nature relies on these beneficial bacteria—billions of them in a single handful of soil—which do the work of decomposition. They reduce dead plants and leaves to nutrients that plants can absorb. Without these miniature ministers of rot and decay, nature's cycle of regeneration ceases to function.

Dedicating one's fields to a single crop (monoculture) is also a problem, apparent to anyone who's ever taken a hike in the woods; Mother Nature doesn't plant things this way. While you might happen upon a forest or meadow where a single species of tree or grass dominates the landscape, there are always other types of vegetation growing nearby. A rich network of plant life attracts insects and animals whose food-seeking behavior helps the ecosystem flourish. A massive field of corn, by contrast, sticks out like a sore thumb. It's a gold-trimmed party invitation to every bug in the vicinity.

"Monoculture leaves you vulnerable," says Scott. "There's always a fear factor looming over your head. If you lose that one crop, you're out of business. So these guys do anything they can to protect their crops." Hence the chemicals or "systemics."

But imagine if a farmer chooses to mimic nature instead. He plants lots of different plants. He throws in some flowers and herbs to attract beneficial insects. And he feeds the soil with well-

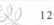

rotted manure and vegetation. "This is the way farmers used to work years ago," Scott says. "We've got a horse stable nearby, so we get all the manure we need, which we turn into compost, and we're always composting our dead plants."

All these rich nutrients mean the fields around Quail Hill Farm are throbbing with life. If aphids attack the tomatoes, lacewings and ladybugs sweep in to devour the pests. Now and then Scott must intervene, and when he does, he uses *Bacillus thuringiensis* (Bt), a microscopic organism applied as a spray or dust that attacks the larvae of pests such as corn borers or Colorado potato beetles. Unlike synthetics, natural pesticides are easily biodegradable. Bt deteriorates rapidly in sunlight.

Each year Scott rotates his crops, never planting the same plant in the spot he planted it the year before. "So many insects are crop-specific," he says. "If I plant in the same spot, they'll say, 'Hey, look, they're growing tomatoes again this year!' and move in. This way, I'm always one step ahead of them."

A single plot of land will wear a couple of different suits in the course of a season. Say Scott plants lettuce and peas in one spot in early spring. When the harvest comes in midsummer, he'll plant "green manure"—a plant known to increase soil fertility—and plow it under when it's high enough. Then he'll plant his fall crops in the same spot. Yields stay high because the soil is always replenished and does not erode. With a mere twenty-five acres, Scott's able to feed two hundred families and still sell excess crops wholesale or make donations to local food pantries. "Doing it this way is a lot more labor-intensive," he says. "There's more hard work, so you need a lot of friends." Quail Hill's CSA is set up to give him those extra hands.

But in other ways, organic farmers are still quite friendless. Banks see them as a bad risk. And conventional farmers who go organic often hide that fact from their neighbors, who fear airborne weed seeds wafting over from the "wilderness" next door. In addition, it typically takes three years to restore the soil—and that long before a farmer can sell crops that are labeled organic. Says Chaskey, "I've heard other farmers say, 'Organic farming is fine on a small scale, but we have to feed the world.' They're forgetting that there are farmers all over the world growing on a small scale and they're feeding billions of people. Look at China."

Given all this, you have to wonder why any farmer would go organic. And yet, more and more are converting every year. About eight thousand farms are certified organic today, and the Organic Farming Research Foundation knows of another twelve to fifteen thousand in the process of converting. Each year sees a 30 percent growth in the number of organic acres. Why the switch? Put simply, organic farming allows farmers to diversify their crops and thus find new markets. Once a farmer is no longer dependent on one crop, he or she enjoys a measure of economic stability. Also, what's good for the land is good for the health of family farmers and workers. In 1996 Vincent Garry at the University of Minnesota Medical School found that birth defects among children of registered pesticide applicators (farmers) were higher than among the regular population. Even nonfarming families in the western half of the state were 85 percent more likely to have birth defects than nonfarming families in the eastern half.

Moreover, organic farming is good future planning. Studies by the Rodale Institute have shown that organic farmland can produce the same yields in an average year and more in times of drought than conventional farms.

EATING ALICE'S WAY

On Shattuck Avenue in Berkeley, California, is a warm, inviting building where diners experience gustatory nirvana. This is the house that Alice Waters built. When she opened Chez Panisse in the early seventies, she insisted that her food be seasonal, local, and organic. Simple as these qualities sound, they were hard to come by in American cuisine at the time. Waters started a trend that affects the kitchen of every fine American restaurant today. All the chefs she trained—a list of Chez Panisse alums reads like a culinary who's who—brought the gospel wherever they went. Waters, a lively, down-to-earth woman, is credited with aiding the resurgence of farmers markets and altering the way many of us eat.

"I suppose organics were somehow in my consciousness from way back," she says. "Because my mother was interested in health food, and I ate things that were different from everybody else in New Jersey in the fifties. Certainly it was part of everybody's thinking in the sixties."

But her true conversion began in France, where as a young American college student she grew accustomed to the fresh daily offerings at local farmers markets. Thus inspired, she began to cook for friends, and the restaurant naturally followed. Trained as a Montessori teacher, she has instead spent her life teaching others to eat well, even outside the walls of the restaurant. Her nonprofit Chez Panisse Foundation has helped fund a garden project at a local prison and is one of the founders of an innovative program at Berkeley's Martin Luther King, Jr., Middle School called the Edible Schoolyard, where students actually grow, cook, and serve their own food. "I want them to learn how to feed themselves in an affordable, delicious, nutritious way," she says. "I would like them to understand and treasure the relationship of food to agriculture, and of food to culture, that the dinner table is a sacred place, a civilizing ritual, and should be important in everyone's life."

We all can benefit from these lessons. Waters believes that the rush to modernity and convenience in the fifties stripped many Americans of their cooking skills. Television ads portrayed kitchen work as drudgery, not pleasure, and the food itself as fuel for growing bodies, not something tasty and nutritious. The good news, she says, is that we can change. "I think it's very easy to do because it's a delicious thing to do," she says, "and because the values are ones that resonate in people's hearts and minds instinctually. It's part of being human. I think they're longing to sit at the table again. And I think they like to be engaged in cooking and serving people they care about."

Alice often hears people saying that they have neither the time nor the money to buy and prepare organic food. She begs to differ. "First of all, in terms of time, I think it's a lot easier to make something of food that is fresh and delicious than it is to doctor up something that is flown in from someplace out of season. I also think that once you get involved in this kind of thinking and shopping, it's so rewarding in other ways that you make time for it, just the way you make time to see a TV show or go to a movie. You meet friends, and the market becomes a meeting place.

"In terms of the money, we have to learn how to cook food that is really tasty using vegetables. I think we don't know how to do that. We're so meat-dependent. But vegetables and grains are certainly affordable food. Polenta for one hundred people is six dollars. People in other countries pay more money for food. We've gotten used to subsidized products, and we don't think we should pay much. But we're certainly willing to pay for cars, houses, and God knows what else. People are getting the message that you may not pay up front for food, but you pay someplace. You pay in your health, you pay in the depletion of natural resources. You're going to pay. It's just whether you want to do it up front and think about the future for our kids, or whether you want to let it go. I want to support the people who are taking care of the land for my kids. And I want to give my dollar directly to the farmer."

That simple transaction may alter the way you think. "I find some of the food so divine that I can't believe it's so inexpensive," Waters says. "When I think about what it takes to grow two dozen radishes, how much time and space, picking them and wrapping them and taking them down there. And you're only selling them for a dollar? That's your whole crop out there. A dollar? Once you get involved with farming, you begin to see what a difficult and unpredictable thing it is. We need those farmers. They're like teachers. We need teachers and farmers, and how can it be we're unwilling to pay for either one?"

GRINGO DOES MEXICAN—BEAUTIFULLY

Like Alice Waters, Rick Bayless was influenced early on by contact with another culture. He was only fourteen years old when he took his first trip outside the United States. His family, who hailed from Oklahoma City, zipped down to Mexico to see the sights of Mexico City and Acapulco. From then on, Bayless recalls, "I was fascinated with Mexico, in love with Mexico. I went every year with high school groups and ended up doing my undergraduate degree in Spanish language and Latin American studies."

He would have gone on to earn a Ph.D. in anthropological linguistics—the study of language and culture—but he stopped mid-dissertation to do what he was clearly born to do: make great food. Rick is descended from four generations of restaurateurs, caterers, and grocers. But while his family served up barbecue, Bayless felt the tug of another cuisine. Today he's hailed as the most inventive chef of Mexican cuisine in the United States. His Chicago restaurants, Frontera Grill and Topolobampo, are consistently ranked among the best in the nation. And millions watch his PBS series, *Mexico: One Plate at a Time,* in which he presents generous helpings of both food and culture.

What his viewers may not know is that Bayless is a zealous supporter of sustainable agriculture. He's a director of the Chef's Collaborative, an association of American chefs devoted to this cause. "With me it's first local, second organic," he says. "I believe that if we save our local farmers, then we have a chance to reform them. But if we let them all go out of business, we have no one to talk to."

His interest in local produce grew during the five years he and his wife, Deann, lived in Mexico, researching his first book. "There's such a different system there that it's almost hilarious to try to compare it with the United States," he says. "I never shopped in a grocery store. I went to markets. When you see these poor, indigenous women who have gone out to the wild and collected these beautiful things"—such as edible mushrooms, plants, and roots—"and they present them like they are jewels for you to buy, there is something moving about that. Of course things collected from the wild are organic. It is so much of the earth itself that I find it incredibly satisfying. The flavor is there, the quality is there, and the uniqueness is there."

Starting out in Chicago in 1987, though, Rick was disappointed to find little organic produce available. But his willingness to search it out and encourage local farmers has led to what is today a remarkable network that goes beyond the traditional relationship between restaurant and purveyor. "We're very close with our farmers," he says. "We have our sous chefs go work on their farms so they understand where the food is coming from. These people are part of our family. They're not our suppliers. They are our partners, and we use those words when we talk to them."

All the food the restaurants serve comes from farms outside Chicago—even in the depths of winter. "If you garden with the seasons, and know how to work the fields, you can extend the season," he says. "We have locally grown produce on our menu twelve months a year. We have invested in these farms. We have literally given them loans so they can build hoop houses"—shelters for crops grown directly in the soil—"and garden all winter."

Some crops, such as spinach, are still wonderful when winter-grown. Tomatoes aren't, so keeping the restaurant stocked with them year-round calls for ingenuity. During the summer, one farmer buys as many organic local tomatoes as he can and freezes them whole. (One year he stockpiled sixteen thousand pounds!) Come winter, he makes a weekly forty-pound delivery to the Frontera kitchens, where the staff whips the iced orbs into sauce. The same goes for fruits, berries, and other irreplaceable summer vegetables. And the taste is still fabulous.

During the summertime Bayless grows herbs, edible flowers, and some small greens in his home garden. Each winter he grows baby greens under grow lights in his basement. Meanwhile, in the basement below his Clark Street restaurants, he's installed a root cellar to keep vegetables such as potatoes, carrots, and garlic cool and fresh. This might sound like a lot of unnecessary trouble, but

Bayless is simply using today's technology to go back to the way things were always done.

For Bayless, the link between farmer and diner is the most important part of the organic movement. "I urge people to get out and try to buy something from an organic grower. Visit their farms, buy from them directly, pick it up at the farm. Visit them on a Sunday afternoon when you're going for a drive in the countryside. You will get an appreciation for the care with which they have grown these things, and your appreciation of that flavor and the beauty of that produce will be that much greater. Once you

- Twenty thousand farmworkers die each year from exposure to chemicals. One million are poisoned but recover.

- Organic farming is the fastest-growing segment of U.S. agriculture, with sales rising 20 percent a year.

- Since 1900, six thousand apple varieties and twenty-three hundred pear varieties have gone extinct due to monoculture farming.

(Source: *Eating to Save the Earth,* Riebel and Jacobsen)

do that, you're going to say, 'Oh! We're *really* preserving community here, and these are people who really care about things.' So supporting organic farmers is really about supporting small communities, caring for the land, and eating in the rhythms of nature.

"The farmers we work with don't have a whole lot of money, but they have a great quality of life. They love what they do, they love the earth, they love their fields, and they love the plants that produce this gorgeous produce. When they bring their produce to us at the restaurant it's like they're bringing us their treasures. They're offering us a little bit of themselves. And that's what we do when we put it down in front of our guests. We're offering them a little bit of ourselves."

What You Can Do

Here are a few ways you and your family can take back control of your food, eat healthfully, and help care for the land.

> *I like to eat organic food, and in fact I grow a lot of it at the house. The vegetables we buy at the market we just wash and wash and wash. I'm not sure I should be saying this, but I always plant a small area of potatoes without any chemicals. By the end of the season, my field potatoes are fine to eat, but any potatoes I pulled today are probably still full of systemics. I don't eat them.*
>
> *—Idaho potato farmer who uses pesticides, quoted in Michael Pollan,* The Botany of Desire

Look for the label. As of October 2002, anyone who sells a product as "organic" must be certified by a USDA-accredited certification agency, such as Oregon Tilth (www.tilth.org). In general, a "certified organic" label is your guarantee that a product was grown, raised, or processed without harmful pesticides, hormones, antibiotics, genetically modified organisms (GMOs), irradiation, or sewage-sludge fertilizers. (There's more stuff that's legal by conventional standards, but I don't want you to lose your appetite.) Processed foods—such as soy milk or a certain brand of highly delicious cookies—are labeled one of three ways:

- "100 percent organic" means all individual ingredients are organic.

- "Organic" means 95 percent of the ingredients are organic.

- "Made with organic ingredients" means at least 70 percent of the ingredients are organic.

Buy local produce in season. The fewer miles a radish must travel from the earth to your mouth, the fewer resources it consumes and the less trash it generates. (In fact, when I'm working in my garden, the trip is literally hand to mouth.) The same is true when you buy a crop in its rightful season. In my opinion, buying local makes the most environmental sense.

- Farmers' markets, coops, and CSAs allow you to buy the food directly from the people who grow or make it. They can answer any questions, and the money stays within the local community. Precious little fuel or packaging has been used to get those scallions into your hot little hands.

Buy organic. Shop at natural-food stores. Large chains such as Wild Oats (www.wildoats.com) or Whole Foods (www.whole foods.com) as well as smaller health-food stores and stands offer a wider range of organic products, albeit from distant locations. This is the perfect place to get produce in winter, when nothing's in season in your area.

Look for organic foods at conventional supermarkets. Most traditional supermarkets now carry a small selection of organic produce and a wide selection of processed organic foods, such as pasta, soy milk, and snacks.

Shop around. Eating for better health or a better planet does not require you to relinquish your hard-earned food-shopping savvy. If you feel that a market is particularly elitist—and admittedly, this happens—look elsewhere. Start by compiling a mental or written list of the organic-food purveyors in your area, and get in the habit of checking in on them when you're in the neighbor-hood. Eventually, you'll narrow your choices to one or two places you like best for variety and service.

Eat lower on the food chain. Producing meat and other animal products taxes our planet unduly. Seven calories of a vegetarian food must be consumed to create a single calorie of animal pro-tein. It takes the equivalent of seventy-eight calories of fuel to cre-ate a single calorie of feedlot beef. When you consciously choose to eat less meat and more grains, vegetables, fruits, and legumes, you are helping reduce the burden of food production on the earth. When you do eat animal proteins, try to stick to organic sources that are hormone- and antibiotic-free by definition. (As you saw earlier, toxins bioaccumulate and become more concen-trated in the bodies of animals. The hormone issue is the chief reason why Europeans refuse to import U.S.-raised beef.) Organic eggs and dairy products are probably already available in your supermarket. You may need to go to a natural-food store for organic meats and poultry. In recent years there's been a movement toward raising cattle hormone- and drug-free on organically grown grass. See the Resources Directory for suppliers.

Farm-raised fish are generally raised using hormones and antibiotics in polluted waters. Try to buy species of wild fish that are not endangered. Check out the Monterey Bay Aquarium site for up-to-date fish news and a list of sustainably harvested fisheries (www.mbayaq.org/cr/seafoodwatch.asp).

Flexatarianism

I'm what you'd call a "flexatarian." I prefer to eat lots of fruits and vegetables, but I'm not averse to eating meat, poultry, and fish from time to time. It depends on the circumstance. I do admire the goals of vegetarians but I've always valued flexibility in eating. If I'm in New Orleans, I'll try gumbo. Or chowder and lobster in Maine. If a business associate is taking me out to dinner, or a friend has graciously prepared a wonderful dinner, I think it's more fun to enjoy the food before me than to scrutinize ingredients. Food *and* friends make the meal.

Consider CSAs. As you saw earlier, Community Supported Agriculture (CSA) is an innovative way to bring fresh organic produce to your table. Popularized in the United States by the late Robin Van En in the mid-eighties, the concept works this way: at the beginning of a growing season, you buy a "share" in a local farmer's harvest. Each week, as the crop comes in, you either drive to the farm to pick it up or the produce is delivered to your neighborhood. The food couldn't be fresher, and you are directly supporting a farming operation. Not all CSAs are organic. Check before you participate. See Local Harvest (www.localharvest.org) or the Robin Van En Center (www.csacenter.org).

Is Eating Organic Expensive?

The price of an organic apple more accurately reflects what cleaner, safer food is worth. Conventional farmers sell a cheaper apple but jeopardize the fruit, their fields, and our health to do it. Society and nature pay the full price later on. Farmers who vow not to use chemicals commit themselves to a pricier way of life. Like neurotic parents, they're constantly employing labor-intensive strategies to keep their charges—and the environment—from harm. The fact is, prices of organic food have dropped considerably as growers have built their markets, and they will continue to do so. Be a consuming pioneer! When Newman's Own Organics first introduced chocolate bars, we had to price them at $2.39. As volume grew we were able to reduce the price to $1.99. If a particular item, like peaches, for example, is too expensive for your budget, you can help by buying finished organic products like peach jam.

Consider co-ops, buying clubs, or delivery services. This option banishes forever the old excuse that organic food is impossible to find. A number of businesses will deliver bulk foods straight to your door. The catch: you must team up with friends and neighbors to meet the dollar minimum (usually starting at three hundred dollars per order). Others, such as Diamond Organics (www.diamondorganics.com), will send fresh produce anywhere in the country overnight. If you go this route, be sure you've exhausted all other local avenues, then choose a business closest to you. Shipping food cross-country is what we're trying to avoid.

See the Resources Directory for names and addresses.

Prioritize your vittles. If you can't switch entirely to organic produce, focus on avoiding the most heavily contaminated fruits and vegetables (see sidebar). Limit your intake of conventionally produced proteins—eggs, dairy products, meats, and poultry, which may contain hormones, antibiotics, and pesticides, along with farm-raised fish, which are often raised in polluted waters using some of the same offenders. When buying full- or high-fat milk, cheese, and yogurt, it is important to buy organic since chemicals lodge in the fat. When you buy conventional produce, wash well or peel. Avoid nonorganic dried fruits because the concentration level of pesticides is much higher and you can't wash them. Choose organic baby food for infants whenever possible because small bodies turn over lots of calories and are thus more vulnerable. And the damage can be to a child's actual *development* rather than "just" health.

Can what we eat come back to haunt us? The evidence here is not conclusive: breast cancer rates in industrial countries have risen 1 percent a year since 1940. Prostate cancer has risen 3.9 percent a year between 1973 and 1991. Sperm counts have dropped about 1 percent a year since 1970 for men in Western countries. Childhood cancer is on the rise. And the age of sexual maturity is declining: in the United States one in seven Caucasian girls and one in two African-American girls start to develop breasts and pubic hair by age eight. Since human physiology is so complex, scientists will always have a tough time identifying the root cause of these problems. Is it food, other things in our environment, or both? No one knows. No matter what we do, we're going to be exposed to dangerous chemicals. Eating organic is a simple and effective way to drastically reduce your body's toxic load and free our land from a significant source of contamination.

The 12 Most Contaminated Fruits and Vegetables

1. Strawberries
2. Bell peppers (from USA and Mexico)*
3. Spinach*
4. Cherries (from USA)
5. Peaches
6. Cantaloupe (from Mexico)
7. Celery
8. Apples
9. Apricots
10. Green beans
11. Grapes (from Chile)
12. Cucumbers

*These vegetables are tied in their ranking.

(Source: Environmental Working Group, compiled from FDA and EPA data)

Avoid overpackaged items when possible. Manufacturing plastic bottles, tin cans, plastic wrap, cardboard boxes—all the stuff we use to package our food—consumes precious fuel, which in turn pollutes the air we breathe. The resulting trash, to the tune of 200 million tons a day, must be landfilled, incinerated, or dumped. Keep this in mind as you do your food shopping. Bulk

Choose Coffee and Chocolate Carefully

Coffee and chocolate consumed in the United States hail from developing nations where both humans and the environment are easily exploited. Officials have actually documented cases of child slavery in African plantations that grow cacao, the tree from which cocoa beans are harvested. It's appalling to think that such practices still exist, but human dignity and sustainable agriculture are both achievable in these markets. Chocolate and coffee labeled "fair-trade certified" ensure that workers were paid a better-than-average wage and the buyer is helping the farmers convert to organic farming. Products labeled "organic" or "shade-grown" have a slightly different meaning. Cacao and coffee grow naturally under the shade of taller trees. But commercial growers have traditionally ignored this natural habitat. They plant the trees in the hot sun, and keep them thriving with fertilizers and pesticides. Yields are higher than they would be under the cool canopy, but eventually the exhausted trees die and must be replaced. "Shade-grown" farming of these two crops helps restore precious habitat for migrating birds, but only the "organic" moniker ensures it was grown without pesticides. Keep an eye out for other fair-trade products such as tea and bananas. See the Resources Directory for good sources of fair-trade coffee and chocolates.

foods are burgeoning these days, and you should have no problem locating dry beans, granola, loose teas, nuts, dried fruits, and whole grains. Choose paper and cardboard—which biodegrade—over plastic cartons and bags. In either case, be sure to reuse bags for other purposes. And try to bring your own bags when you shop. At home, reduce or eliminate use of disposable items such as paper towels, napkins, and Styrofoam plates. Use cloth, glass, and regular dishware whenever feasible. Choose reusable containers for lunch items to avoid individually wrapped foods.

Dine out simply and organically. Try to reduce food packaging and waste in meals you eat away from home. Most of us keep a mug at work, but why not a set of cutlery and a cloth napkin or two? (I know one woman who carries a set in her purse to avoid using plastic forks, spoons, and knives.) A camper's bottle or thermos means never having to buy another drink on the go, or, if you do buy coffee on the run, you can use your own thermos or insulated cup. When you're dining out or planning a catered event, consider patronizing restaurants that support organic farmers. For a list of great places to eat, see the Chef's Collaborative (www.chefnet.com/cc2000).

Rachel Carson: Mother of the Environmental Movement

The greatest forces for change are often the most unassuming people. Rachel Carson, a zoologist who grew up in rural Pennsylvania, is credited with sparking the environmental movement that lasts to this day. Carson was a government scientist who wrote and edited radio scripts and other reports for the U.S. Fish and Wildlife Service. On the side she wrote nature articles and books about ecology and the sea. In 1962 she published *Silent Spring*, a scathing indictment of wanton pesticide use in postwar America. Chapter after chapter, she described how government and private agencies sprayed chemicals to control insects—only to have the applications backfire, killing pets, livestock, and wild animals. Humans were next, she warned, because cancer and other ills would be the inevitable result of such reckless policies. "It is our alarming misfortune that so primitive a science has armed itself with the most modern and terrible weapons," she wrote, "and that in turning them against the insects it has also turned them against the earth." Sadly, she herself died of breast cancer in 1964, but not before millions had heard her message.

ONE LAST WORD . . .

One of the "sweetest" phone calls we got at the office of Newman's Own Organics in recent years came from Ray Martin. He and his wife, Mindy, recently opened the Fair Scoop, a small ice cream business in nearby Fairfax, California, and were insisting on making all-organic ice cream. It's easier said than done. Most mom-and-pop ice cream shops in this country mix their own

Organic Wine and Beer

What could be more organic, you might think, than those two ancient beverages, beer and wine? But these days harmful pesticides and herbicides are de rigeur even in the world's hops and grape crops. In the United States a tiny number of companies brew beer with organically grown hops, but those offerings can be tough to find. You'll have better luck locating "organic wine" (from organic grapes, no sulfites) or wine labeled "organically grown" (from organic grapes, with sulfites added as a preservative). In recent years California's winemakers have been toying with a shift to sustainable agriculture.

Fetzer Vineyards, which buys about 2 percent of the grapes crushed in California each year, has decided to take the plunge. The company is now mandating that all its grape suppliers go organic by 2010. Fetzer already sells an "organically grown" line under the label Bonterra (www.bonterra.com), but this move means four other Fetzer lines (www.fetzer.com) will eventually go organic. The decision, says Paul Dolan, Fetzer's winemaker-president, comes after careful experimentation at Fetzer's vineyards in Hopland, California. "Organic grapes taste better," he says. "So we think it's important to do this. We want to make a difference in agriculture around the world. Other people will see us do this, so they'll do it too." Fetzer is already something of an environmental paragon; they make barrels locally at their own cooperage and use electric factory vehicles, kenaf labels with soy-based inks, recycled glass bottles, and real beeswax to seal corks.

Not all companies will take it that far, but any positive change is to be applauded. "I think you really have to believe in a sustainable lifestyle," says Morgan Wolaver, whose beer (www.wolavers.com) is one of the few organic brews available in the United States. "That's really what it's all about. Even our T-shirts are printed on organic cotton."

A word on buying: you can order organic wine and beer online, but shipping laws vary from state to state. It may be better to simply inquire at your local liquor store, or shop at one of the large natural-food-store chains. See the Resources Directory for more information.

batches in a back room, using a premixed base and ingredients such as nuts, berries, and chocolate chips that they buy from a central distributor.

The distributor in the Martins' area didn't "do" organic, so they had to look elsewhere. They buy their milk-cream-sugar base

---

Raising Organic Kids

Organic fruits and veggies should taste the same as (or better than) conventional produce, so you won't get an argument there from the peanut gallery. But if you're making an effort to eat more healthfully—that is, cutting back on sweets and refined and processed foods—your kids might well gripe if they're already hooked on the stuff. Stock your kitchen with whole-food snack choices such as organic dried fruit, popcorn, and nuts. If you simply must have sweets and soft drinks, check out the offerings at a supermarket such as Wild Oats or Whole Foods.

It's never too soon to teach some basic consumer skills when shopping with your children. Have them help you read labels for nutritional and unit-pricing information. ("How much does that cost per pound?" you might ask. "How many servings are included, realistically?") Ask them to help you look for products bearing the "certified organic" label. When you shop at a farmers market, consider letting them pick their favorite produce, ask the farmer questions, and make the transaction. You might also involve your kids in the kitchen. Allow them to help prepare meals or prepare them on their own. Your enthusiasm and praise will reinforce their attitudes toward healthful food. Keep in mind that the good habits they develop now will put them on the right track for the rest of their lives.

---

from an organic creamery, and they make weekly pickups at local farms and purveyors to get fresh strawberries and other ingredients. We were happy to supply them with Newman O's for their Cookies & Cream ice cream. Needless to say, this is a lot of extra work for the Martins, but they don't mind a bit.

"This is something I believe in," Ray says. "No hormones and no pesticides makes sense to me. Farmers have grown food like

The Wrap Rap

Most of us buy scads of plastic wrap and foil to wrap foods, store stuff in the fridge, and cook in microwaves. We use it once and toss it. Why not do what folks did before foil and plastic wrap existed? Store the food in glass dishes with glass lids. If you don't have any, improvise. Use a bowl with a dinner or dessert plate on top of it. If the bowl you're trying to cover is too big for any of these options, you have to ask yourself, Why am I trying to store something the size of an aircraft carrier in my fridge? It's better and safer to reduce food to smaller sizes anyway: a leftover turkey carcass is an invitation to bacteria, even if kept in the fridge. Cut the bird up and store it in smaller containers.

that for thousands of years, and it was fine. The last sixty to eighty years we've been doing it another way, and it doesn't seem to be for the better. It's questionable to put stuff like that in someone's food."

I'd like to think that we all feel the same way, no matter who we are. Parents in the kitchen, steaming or stirring or chopping, think of the children who will shortly come to the table. The boyfriend thinks of his date. The great chefs think of their diners. The grandmother baking cookies daydreams of her grandchildren. And some years back, trussing that bird for Thanksgiving, I thought of that stubborn father whom I love, and love to tease.

At the heart of it, food *is* love and every meal is a thanksgiving. We all know this, but we don't always take time to think about it. The organic movement is teaching us to cherish food just as we cherish the people to whom we serve it.

CHAPTER 2

TRANSPORTATION

Whither goest thou, America, in thy shiny car in the night?
—Jack Kerouac, *On the Road*

Transportation is a tricky subject when it comes to the environment. Let me come clean and admit up front that I love cars. The nicer and faster, the better. In fact, I think everyone should own a Porsche—if they promise to drive it only on Saturdays and to take public transportation the rest of the time!

There's plenty of justification for such a crazy idea. Consider the "value" of a fancy car. The same amount of energy is used to build and maintain a Porsche as a Toyota. The Porsche is certainly more fun to drive. And someday, if you are reaching for soy chai during a turn and wrap the car around a tree, the parts continue to retain their value at the wrecking yard.

Okay, this argument didn't work on my father, either.

The realities of getting around this planet do pose a problem. Even if you live in a city, public transportation isn't always appealing. It can be convenient and efficient for a daily commute, but striking off on your own at the wheel of your own car is a privilege that Americans won't easily give up. If we agree that the private auto, with its convenience and great sound system, won't disappear anytime soon, then we must build cars so efficiently that they are no longer the biggest single contributor of carbon dioxide in our air. Not to mention the way oil pollutes our waterways, and how our need for it distorts our politics.

Amory Lovins, the top energy expert at the Rocky Mountain Institute, has pioneered an initiative to design a new breed of car. Instead of running on gasoline, it would use hydrogen gas, the most abundant element in the universe. In theory, the car's exhaust would be a harmless, much needed substance: water vapor. The car would also sport regenerative brakes—that is, every time you brake, you're generating additional power to run the electric motor. These cars would also be very quiet, which brings me to another confession: I do like the sound of a well-tuned exhaust note. It must be from spending time with my dad at the racetrack.

Most of the major car manufacturers are now experimenting with hydrogen fuel cells. California's strict auto-emissions legislation is forcing their hand. Elsewhere, drivers are already getting around town in electric cars or cars powered by natural gas. But everyone, including the players who largely control the game, concedes that hydrogen is the way to go. Bill Ford, chairman of Ford Motor Company, recently said, "I believe fuel cells will finally end the one-hundred-year reign of the internal-combustion engine." It may sound unbelievable, but our beloved four-stroke combustion engine just might become obsolete in that hydrogen economy. No one can say just when that will be. The brains behind it say there's still a way to go.

On the Road to Carvana

To get around in Basalt, Colorado, Jon Fox-Rubin drives a little Subaru, which he sometimes shares with his wife. It's a good car, nothing fancy about it, but every time he's behind the wheel Jon can't help thinking of the car of his dreams, a car he and his team are inventing.

Jon is a mechanical engineer and the CEO of Hypercar, Inc., the company designing technology that will one day end up on American roads. He counts as Hypercar's clients some of the biggest automakers in the world. They know the era of gasoline is coming to a close, and they're looking to Hypercar for solutions.

"They'll look just like today's cars," he says. "Maybe a little more aero, a little more European, if I can say that. They'll be the same size as today's cars, fit into today's infrastructure—and eventually they will be environmentally benign."

One of the secrets of making this car work is replacing the heavy steel of auto bodies with composite materials—the same tough carbon fibers used to make skis, fishing rods, snowboards, bikes, and other sports equipment. That switch will help reduce by half the weight of any car on the road today. Automakers have known for years that they could build a safe car this way, but composites haven't been affordable in automotive volumes, that is, hundreds of thousands of auto bodies per year. As a design element, though, there's nothing flimsy about carbon fiber. Race cars and high-performance aircraft are built of the stuff.

Since the lighter frames require less fuel to propel them, these cars can get by on lighter drive systems and lighter engines. You wouldn't notice much of a difference if you saw one of these prototype hydrogen cars on the road today. But you'd feel it in your wallet when you pulled up to the pump. Such hydrogen vehicles "will go three hundred thirty miles on seven and a half pounds of hydrogen," says Jon. "That's the equivalent of 3.3 gallons of gasoline." To translate that into English, it's like getting ninety-nine miles to the gallon in a modern-day car.

I'd hop behind the wheel of one of these cars this instant if I could, but Jon says I'll have to wait. It's still expensive to extract hydrogen from sources such as natural gas. And gas stations would have to be retrofitted to pump the new juice. Still, in five to ten years people who work in airports, police departments, post offices, mass-transit systems, and warehouses will be getting around in the car that spews steam, not smog. A little later, the technology that's perfected in those arenas will end up on a car lot near you.

I don't think we'll be disappointed. Until now, fuel-efficient cars have been synonymous with teensy vehicles. The folks at Hypercar have no intention of letting it stay that way. "Everyone I tell about Hypercars falls in love with the idea," Jon says. "We all live in the mountains, we get snow, and everyone around here drives SUVs. People love the environment, so they're in this perpetual-conflict situation. I think that's why they like our approach. They see it as the coming of a guilt-free sport utility vehicle."

Sign me up.

On Muscle and Sunbeams

Have you ever listened to John Denver's music about the majestic mountains of Colorado—of eagles soaring against a backdrop of blue sky, puffy clouds, and mountain streams? Okay, maybe this will date me, but when I was thirteen I was involved in a documentary about birds of prey, featuring John Denver and naturalist Morley Nelson, called *The Eagle and the Hawk.* The goal of the film was to teach the public about the ecological importance of falcons, hawks, eagles, and all birds of prey—and to discourage people from shooting them, which was a big problem at the time.

This early experience didn't make me a country-music fan, but it did foster my inborn envy of creatures who share the world with us. I was entranced by the speed of the peregrine falcon. I've kept an eye on the sky ever since, and have trained and hunted with many different birds of prey. This hobby, falconry, was once called the sport of kings. I call it the sport of fools, since that's what I'm sure I looked like running through the fields of California artichokes chasing my birds. The grace of these creatures, however—both hunter and prey—is a beautiful example of nature's efficient design.

Paul MacCready understood this. As a boy growing up in Connecticut in the 1920s and 1930s, he collected butterflies and moths. Dyslexic and kind of shy, Paul spent most of his time alone, trying to build model planes and other flying machines out of balsa wood. In college his fascination with fuel-free flight inspired him to take up flying gliders.

Paul eventually went into the weather-modification business.

He was going to be a high-tech rainmaker, using his know-how to help farmers irrigate their land. The business never really took off, but Paul got a reputation for building his way out of any thorny engineering problem. Here's a good one: in the 1950s, Paul and his fellow scientists were having a devil of a time studying rainstorms. Every plane or balloon they flew in a storm ended up pummeled by chunks of ice. So Paul designed and built an armored airplane. No one had ever seen such a thing before.

By the mid-seventies, Paul was a grown man with a family. Looking for some extra cash, he heard about a man in England who was offering a prize to anyone who could build a human-powered aircraft. The Kremer Prize, as it was called, had gone unclaimed for twenty years.

Nights and weekends, Paul and some friends built the *Gossamer Condor,* a wondrous aluminum-and-plastic aircraft with ninety-six-foot wings that flew as its pilot pedaled away in the cockpit. And with it he won the prize.

In 1981 he built the world's first solar-powered airplane. Later he dreamed up a solar-powered automobile, a huge solar flier for NASA called Helios, and a working model of a pterodactyl for an IMAX film. No wonder the American Society of Mechanical Engineers dubbed him "the Engineer of the Century."

About a decade ago Paul and his scientists teamed up with General Motors to design the first mass-market electric car. Electric cars run on a rechargeable battery, and though the energy to charge them still comes from a power plant, such cars eliminate harmful "street-level" emissions. Futurists and environmentalists have crowed about such a vehicle for years, and though a number of small, grass-roots car companies do sell them, until recently Detroit has ignored the concept. Electrics have two tall hurdles to overcome: they need powerful batteries and easily accessible charging stations. For this reason, GM's EV1 didn't really take off.

Industry critics say the GM venture was a foolhardy one, but there's still plenty to learn from the experiment. The car Paul built looks like something Batman would drive—it's the most streamlined vehicle on the road today.

These days, when Paul gives talks, his message is part engineering, part environmentalism. Everywhere he goes, he gives young engineers this advice: do more with less. Mother Nature is the first and finest engineer. The blueprint for any animal—a cheetah, a dolphin, a bumblebee, a human—is perfect because nature abhors waste.

The lessons Paul learned have influenced a new generation of fuel-efficient hybrid-electric cars.

About "Hybrid" Vehicles

Technically speaking, a hybrid is any machine that combines two or more sources of power. Detroit's new vehicles marry time-tested gasoline engines with electric motors and rechargeable batteries. The result is a sophisticated car with reduced tailpipe emissions and superior mileage. These cars run on gas just like ordinary cars. You fill them at the pump as you normally do—you just won't be filling up that often. That's because the car uses fuel

Hybrid Cars Now Available

	MPG (HIGHWAY/CITY)	SEATS	NOTES
Ford Escape HEV	40/29 automatic*	5+	first hybrid SUV; 450 to 550 miles on a tank of gas
Honda Civic hybrid	51/46 automatic	5	40 percent better gas mileage than conventional Civic sedan
Honda Insight	57/56 automatic	2	first U.S.–made hybrid; best mileage of all four
Toyota Prius	52/45 automatic	5	0 to 60 in 14 seconds; made of 90 percent recyclable materials

Hybrid Cars in the Works

	MODEL	YEAR
Ford	Explorer	2005+
General Motors	Saturn SUV	2004
	Chevy pickup	2004
	Chevy Suburban	2005
Daimler-Chrysler	Dodge Ram pickup	2005
	Mercedes S-class	2006

*Models with standard transmission also available

(Source: U.S. Department of Energy: www.fueleconomy.gov)

GM's EV1 (www.gmev.com) is still on the roads in California and Arizona, but Saturn dealerships are no longer taking new leases on them. If you're determined to own an electric vehicle, you might consider one of the fun, peppy cars released by Ford's Think Mobility group (www.thinkmobility.com) or the new Rav4 released by Toyota (www.rav4ev.toyota.com). You can also convert your current car to an electric, or buy an EV from a smaller, independent company. The Electric Vehicle Association of American (www.evaa.org) is the best place to start. On average, a car like the EV1 gets about 75 to 130 miles on a single charge. (It takes six to eight hours to charge its nickel metal hydride battery. An alternative lead-acid battery recharges in two and a half to six hours but gets only 55 to 95 miles per charge.) Smaller vehicles, such as Ford's City, muster a 50-mile range after a four- to six-hour charge. These ranges are still ideal for commuting and running errands—and you'll never catch a whiff of gasoline while refueling.

more intelligently and relies upon the electric motor for backup power. When you're stopped at a light, the car switches off its gas engine and runs on the electric motor. The car slips through the air with little resistance thanks to its light, aerodynamic design. Best of all, you'll never have to plug it in. Each time you brake, the car charges the electric motor.

My mother is hardly the car buff in our family. Pa and I take that prize. But Ma was the first in her neighborhood to insist on getting a hybrid-electric car, which she happily uses to run errands. I drive it now and then when I'm home visiting. It'll never win a drag race, but it gets phenomenal mileage.

What You Can Do

Until we're all whizzing around in Hypercars, here are a few ways to conserve transportation fuel.

Streamline your car. Cars travel best when they reduce "drag"—the amount of air whipping over the car. Flags, roof racks, bicycles, and open windows all slow you down and guzzle fuel.

Observe the speed limit. You are not Mario Andretti. You are not even my father. Stick to the posted limit, and you'll keep your car functioning optimally.

Keep it smooth. Stomping on the gas and slamming on the brakes is the surest way to waste fuel. Jackrabbits make poor drivers. Keep your speed consistent.

Idle not. If you're not going anywhere, or if you're stuck in traffic, shut the car off. You're already wasting time. Why waste gas too?

Take care of your car. An old friend used to say, "Everything in life is maintenance. You maintain your friendships. You maintain your health. You maintain your car." (Actually, this guy maintained only his car, but that's another story.) Stick to the suggested

- Cars and light trucks consume 40 percent of U.S. oil and cough up 20 percent of the nation's CO_2.

- The average car emits 70 tons of CO_2 in its lifetime, the average SUV about 100 tons.

- The average U.S. car gets 27.5 miles per gallon, small trucks 20.7. If we raised fuel-efficiency standards to 45 mpg and 34 mpg, we'd cut CO_2 pollution by 600 tons and save $45 billion at the pump each year.

maintenance schedule, and treat yourself to an oil change every three thousand miles. Your owner's manual will give you specific guidelines for top performance.

If your car has the option, shift into overdrive. You don't need all the power your engine cooks up when you're driving at a constant speed on a flat road. Shifting into overdrive allows the engine to run slower, maintains speed, and uses less fuel.

Keep your tires inflated properly. Your car has to work harder when its tires are under- or overinflated. Check the air regularly with a pressure gauge.

Carpool, or take the bus or train. The logic is simple. One person in a car gets twenty miles per gallon. If two people ride in the same car, you've saved twenty "passenger miles" per gallon. Buses, which typically hold fifty passengers, can get one thousand passenger miles in a single ride. Trains? Anyone here good at math? Anyway, you get the idea.

Hustle locally on muscle. A 160-pound person burns 317 calories on a one-hour walk. Walking is great exercise. If time is the issue, ride a bike. A bike outfitted with baskets or saddlebags can carry a lot more stuff than any two hands.

Rent an environmentally friendly car when traveling. EV Rental Cars (www.evrental.com) offers electric, natural-gas, and hybrid vehicles in twelve cities across the United States. (Most are in California; other cities include Pittsburgh, Washington, D.C., and Phoenix.) This is one of the best ways to test-drive a vehicle if you're considering taking the plunge. According to EV Rental, the benefits of driving these cars go beyond the fact that you're conserving fuel; sometimes it's a selfish delight. Consider: drivers who are traveling alone can still use the car-pool lanes in California, Arizona, Virginia, and Georgia. Charging electric vehicles is still free (locations are provided on maps from the rental agency), and you can fill the tank in a natural-gas car for about three to four dollars. Hybrids get about forty to sixty miles per gallon.

If you're buying a car, make fuel efficiency a high priority. Each year, the American Council for an Energy-Efficient Economy (ACEE) crunches the numbers on all production-line vehicles and ranks them according to efficiency. You can check out the greenest and "meanest" cars for free on their website (www .greenercars.com). A print edition of their guide, or an online access to their data, can be had for a small subscription fee. It's well worth it if you're in the market for a car.

One Last Word . . .

Keep it all in perspective. At the end of the day, the infrastructure of this nation is built to enshrine the American automobile. In most cities and suburbs in America, bicycling to the mall—a trip that could entail riding on two major freeways, over three overpasses, down dangerous off-ramps—would be absolutely nuts. Don't be too hard on yourself. The goal is to *reduce* fuel consumption and planet-warming emissions. The measures listed in this chapter are, to a certain extent, buying us time until the world is running on sunbeams and hydrogen. When that day comes, we'll still need cars. But then you and I can take the Porsche out every day of the week.

CHAPTER 3

ENERGY AND WATER

*What's the use of a house if you haven't got
a tolerable planet to put it on?*
—HENRY DAVID THOREAU

ENERGY

In the summer of 1985 I was standing on a large granite rock that was covered in lichens and surrounded by wild blueberries and stunted pine trees. I had just purchased three acres of raw, undeveloped New England land. My plan was to live there, with the birch trees, chickadees, and black flies.

The air carried a hint of salt from Frenchman Bay, about three miles to the west as the crow flies. The nearest potable water or electric outlet was about as far. In the optimistic mind of a young college student, however, water and electricity presented only a small obstacle to what was to be a Thoreauvian summer in Maine. My vision included a small garden of red-tipped lettuce, snow peas, and peppers set against the backdrop of canvas from a twenty-foot-diameter tepee.

I soon learned that tepee poles are about thirty-two feet long, and a five-gallon jug of water weighs about thirty-eight pounds. And the light from an oil lamp casts a romantic hue but struggles against a moonless Maine night.

As my college professor William Drury would say, "If something is challenging your perspective, or making you uncomfortable, pay attention, you are about to learn something."

The joy of owning land, setting up the tepee, and feeling connected to a specific place was incredibly satisfying, grounding—almost tribal. But my first real lesson about water and energy—luxuries that previously were only a faucet and light switch away—arrived abruptly as the batteries in my flashlight died my first night. The absence of basic comforts was sobering, and fostered an appreciation for what most of the world's population faces as a daily reality.

I had elected to face these challenges but did so knowing that technologies were available that could bring some comfort to my primitive dwelling. I was armed with a copy of the Real Goods catalog (which had gone from coffee-table fixture to a resource on photovoltaic panels, batteries, solar showers, and efficient cookstoves) as my guide—and an excellent fly swatter!

Real Goods is today's largest renewable-energy retailer. Its founder, John Schaeffer, graduated from Berkeley in 1971, then he and his radical buddies headed for the rural hills of Mendocino County, California, to be one with nature. Lucky for me, they had a thirteen-year head start on the discovery that untrammeled nature did not come with lights or running water.

John didn't let that get him down. His idealism was leavened by his entrepreneurship. It wasn't long before he was driving back to civilization, loading up his Volkswagen bus with hand tools, water pipes, generators, lightbulbs, fertilizer, and so on, and hauling it all back to the hills to sell to his fellow hippies. Tired of squinting by the light of their kerosene lanterns, his friends snapped up his common-sense provisions, and in 1978 John opened a kind of New Age general store. He crammed the place with everything one needed to live in the woods: wind turbines, woodstoves, chicken wire, tough outdoor clothing, and scads of how-to books.

After opening his third California store, John began selling his products by mail. Real Goods was the first company to sell solar-power supplies to the public. Its capable staff technicians dispensed advice by phone to legions of people who longed to live off the grid—independent of public power-supply lines. One of the wackiest things they ever sold was an instant "Off-the-Grid Kit" that consisted of a huge tent, an electric motorcycle, a solar-power system, a composting toilet, a water heater, solar mosquito repellant, and a solar hat fan, delivered and installed anywhere in the world for $19,995.

My tepee sported a very basic system: one 120-watt photovoltaic panel providing enough energy to charge a deep-cycle marine battery. My homestead appliances included a single 12-volt, 25-watt bulb, a toaster, a radio, and a 12-inch black-and-white television. The Maine sky had enough sunshine to power my summer and fill the bushes with tiny sweet wild blueberries. I can remember watching the evening news while throwing a sneaker at an intruding raccoon who couldn't resist either the blueberries or Peter Jennings.

Real Goods customers have changed from the old days. "It used to be that we were wackos," John tells us. "But now pretty much anyone is smart to convert to solar power. The cost of solar is coming down every year, and the electricity rates are going up. So it's almost a no-brainer. It used to be that we were radicals who were making a political statement. It's not a political issue anymore. People today understand what solar can do for us. They know it decreases reliance on foreign oil. They switch for environmental reasons. They do it because they feel good doing it."

John notices that business picks up whenever a natural or political disaster reveals vulnerable cracks in the American way of life. In the seventies and eighties, it was the Three Mile Island nuclear accident, the energy crisis, and the taking of the U.S. Embassy in Iran. Today Americans are no strangers to water shortages, "boil-water" emergencies, and sewer leaks that contaminate beaches and rivers. Frequent energy shortages and the September 11 tragedy are encouraging people to look for ways to reduce our oil dependency.

It's still costly to convert an entire home to solar power. But homeowners are discovering they can save energy simply by installing compact fluorescent lightbulbs, using rechargeable batteries to power small electronics, and better insulating their home and windows. For new-home construction in a remote location, solar power is often less expensive than installing power lines and poles. Anyone interested in a used tepee?

The American home, with its abundance of electric appliances, is the perfect voting booth for social change. In this chapter we'll show you how to make a dent in your pattern of energy use. You'll realize, as I have, that lower energy bills are just the beginning of the rewards for treading lightly, because the more you know, the less you need.

Tackle what you can of the suggestions here. In time you'll find yourself conserving without trying. Consciously or unconsciously, you will end up doing more with less. Washing will take less time. Your machines will serve you better. And you'll pocket some savings each month when the utility bills arrive.

By simplifying your life in these areas, you may find you have more time to spend with family and friends. So sit outdoors with them on a night lit only by fireflies. Read to your kids by candlelight. On beautiful, sunny days, throw open the windows and shades and let in natural light.

The Trouble with Electricity

Generating electricity—extracting power out of coal and other fossil fuels or out of nuclear fission—is the leading cause of air pollution in the United States. In the U.S. about two thirds of all sulfur dioxide and one fourth of all nitrogen oxide in the air you breathe comes from electric-power generation that relies on burning fossil fuels. Power plants spew harmful chemicals and particles, described below, that cause, conservatively, one hundred thousand deaths in the United States each year.

- Sulfur dioxide, the chief cause of acid rain, kills plants, defaces manmade structures, and harms people's lungs. Asthma sufferers are especially susceptible to health problems caused by sulfur dioxide, which can trigger attacks.

 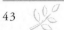

- Mercury, which lodges in the fatty tissue of humans, livestock, and wild animals, causes liver damage and birth defects.

- Nitrogen oxide, the number one ingredient in smog, also causes pulmonary disorders in animals.

- Toxic soot, which settles on crops, waterways, gardens, and windowsills, is inhaled and is associated with cancer, asthma, heart and lung diseases.

- Carbon dioxide is the chief cause of global warming. Currently power plants emit about one ton of CO_2 per person in the United States each year. Combined with CO_2 from other sources—cars, trucks, planes, even the smallest campfire—it adds up. The United States has 5 percent of the world's population but produces *25 percent* of the earth's CO_2.

- Radioactive waste, the dangerous debris of nuclear-power plants, causes cancer and birth defects. By-products of uranium and plutonium can linger in the atmosphere for thousands of years. Improperly stored or carelessly handled, they easily contaminate land, waterways, and entire nations for eons. Fallout from the 1986 meltdown at Chernobyl in the former Soviet Union spread as far west as England. Hardest hit, of course, are those who live closest to the site. Generations of people are destined to eat tainted crops off ruined land, suffer diseases like leukemia and thyroid cancer, and witness the birth of children with heartbreaking deformities.

EARTH'S TWO BIGGEST PROBLEMS

The Greenhouse Effect

The earth is choking to death on greenhouse gases. Chief among these is carbon dioxide, the naturally occurring gas that is the chief by-product of animal respiration and combustion. Plants drink in CO_2 and exhale precious oxygen. But ever since the first time a human burned a tree, human actions have consistently altered this delicate reciprocal relationship. Today, as vast quantities of fossil fuels—coal, oil, and gas—are incinerated, the resulting CO_2 is pumped into the atmosphere—about six billion tons worldwide at the current rate. (A quarter of it comes from the United States.) These gases act like greenhouse windows; they let the sun's heat in but don't let it out. As a result, the earth's temperatures have risen about 1 degree Fahrenheit over the last century. If we don't act to reduce our CO_2 emissions, temperatures in the United States could rise 3 to 11 degrees on average in the next one hundred years.

Kyoto Protocols Working

While our continent tilts ever more rightward, rewarding the energy industry with fewer restrictions, the European Union is almost halfway to achieving the emissions reductions mandated by the Kyoto Protocol on climate change. According to the European Environmental Agency, the fifteen-nation bloc has successfully decreased emissions of carbon dioxide and other greenhouse gases to 3.5 percent below 1990 levels; under Kyoto, EU levels must drop to 8 percent below 1990 levels by 2008–2012. Will our government ever catch on that climatic change isn't just a political issue? Voice your political opinion by sending an e-mail to your elected officials. You can do so easily by going to www.congress.org.

A one-degree rise doesn't sound like much, but scientists have noticed erratic weather patterns that may be the result of increased precipitation in the atmosphere. In Alaska the average temperature has risen seven degrees over the last thirty years. Entire villages are being moved due to rising water levels. Homes are sinking because the ground, which used to remain frozen year-round, is melting. And insects that used to be killed off each winter are surviving to decimate forests. In the Alps, glaciers have shrunk 50 percent since 1900. In Antarctica a major ice shelf recently lost an ice chunk of unprecedented size, as large as Connecticut. A pattern of devastating floods and droughts has established itself in the United States and elsewhere. And infectious diseases—such as West Nile virus—are appearing in North America for the first time.

Scientists caution people against seizing upon local weather patterns, which are naturally variable, as evidence of global warming. But I suspect all of us can think of local changes in weather patterns we'd like to see investigated. Each winter the Aspetuck River, which flowed through my childhood backyard, would freeze solid and provide an ice-skating highway for all the neighborhood kids. Now the river hasn't frozen solid enough for skating in twenty years. Coincidence?

Ozone Depletion

Like a pair of cool shades protecting your eyes, the ozone layer is a chemical shield six to thirty miles above the earth that protects all life from the damaging effects of the sun's ultraviolet (UV-B) rays. Ozone, or O_3, consists of three oxygen atoms. Human use of chemicals has resulted in tons of chlorine gas being released into the atmosphere. Chlorine attacks ozone molecules and shreds the three oxygen atoms into O_2 (a molecule of breathable air) and a single oxygen atom. As ozone disappears, more UV-B rays bombard the earth, leaving all life—human, animal, plants—vulnerable.

Currently the ozone layer above Antarctica fluctuates between 40 to 70 percent of its pre-1980 levels. By September 1999 the hole over the South Pole had grown to two and a half times the size of Europe. The increased sunlight that gets through can decimate forests, crops, and marine life. In 1991 the U.S. Environmental Protection Agency (EPA) predicted that over the next fifty years twelve million Americans will contract skin cancer and two hundred thousand will die from malignant melanoma. Under the direction of the UN, nations are working to halt the release of ozone-depleting substances.

Fossil Fuels:
How Many Years Have We Got?

The most optimistic analysts—the petroleum industry itself—estimate that the earth's remaining oil reserves will last us another fifty to one hundred years, tops. Proven natural-gas reserves will last sixty years, coal another two hundred. The Great Unsaid: accessing remaining oil will become increasingly more expensive and pose greater risks to the environment. For now the issue is not availability but degradation of the planet. Poor old Earth can't afford another fifty, sixty, or two hundred years of CO_2 being pumped into the atmosphere. Incidentally, clean, free energy from the sun will last another five billion years.

Renewable Energy

Where will the energy of the future come from? From the sun, wind, earth, and water, of course. These resources are all renewable; as long as the earth thrives, they'll be abundant. Besides solar and wind power, humans can harvest geothermal energy (from the earth's own heat and lava); tidal power (from the twice-daily changes in sea levels); hydropower (from small water dams that don't harm surroundings); and cogeneration (the production of two forms of energy from one process, as when excess steam from manufacturing is used to generate electricity for the factory or to sell to a power company). Renewable energies could easily become the world's great economic equalizer. Once the infrastructures are built, the raw materials are forever free. Here's a look at the two leaders in alternative energies.

Solar Power

In one day the sun bombards the earth with more energy than the earth's population would consume in twenty-seven years. Today the sun supplies less than 1 percent of the United States' electricity consumption. As the cost of fossil fuels rises, power companies will most likely increase their solar-power facilities and supplement them with investments in wind power. In the meantime, homes can be designed more efficiently to exploit the sun's warmth—with large windows pointing to the south, tile and cement floors to absorb and radiate heat, and windows that retain heat at night. Though it's still quite expensive to retrofit an entire home for solar power, it's now economically feasible to meet a portion of your electricity, hot-water, or space-heating needs with a "grid intertie" system.

Living off the Grid

Wouldn't it be sweet to unplug your entire home from the power company? Many Americans have done just that, replacing "store-bought" energy with power generated on their own property. Christopher Borton and Linda Welsh live in the woods outside Butte, Montana, without a drop of juice from the local power authority. They harvest the sun's rays with photovoltaics, capture passing breezes with wind turbines, and store it all in a battery bank the size of a small closet. "Wind and solar really complement each other," says Chris. "When the weather's bad and there's not much sun, the wind usually picks up. And when the weather clears, the sun comes out." They're hardly roughing it; this hybrid system powers their 5,000-square-foot home and a 1,400-square-foot guest house.

Here's how it works: contractors install photovoltaic arrays on your property, along with a control panel that automatically switches to the power company when necessary. If, by chance, you generate more solar energy in a billing cycle than you need, power companies are required by recent "net-metering" laws to credit your account. In some markets, power companies also offer rebates to those who retrofit their homes. Check with your energy supplier to see if such a program exists in your area.

Wind Power

Wind is now the fastest-growing form of energy in the United States. It currently supplies only .3 percent of U.S. energy, but that figure will climb to 6 percent by 2020. (Some days I wish the United States could move faster.) Denmark now meets 15 percent of its power needs with those graceful, spinning propellers and plans to reach 50 percent by 2020. Germany and Sweden are close behind. Ireland is building a two-hundred-turbine farm—the world's largest—off its Emerald Coast. Upon completion, this single site will generate 10 percent of that nation's electricity. In the United States, a New England firm recently proposed building a 170-turbine farm off the coast of Cape Cod. Environmentalists worry that the forty-story turbines will devastate flocks of migrating birds, harm fisheries, and scare off tourists who now flock to the Cape. Builders feel confident they can design turbines that minimize environmental impact.

WATER

Water, water, everywhere,
Nor any drop to drink.
—SAMUEL TAYLOR COLERIDGE

Rural Connecticut is lush and green in the summer, with frequent afternoon thundershowers and countless streams meandering toward brackish marshes. Neighborhood lawns are golf-course green tended with armies of sprinkler systems. My childhood home in Westport, Connecticut, had a sprinkler system that drew water from the Aspetuck River, my backyard playground. Water, it seemed, was in endless supply. The river was waist deep, full of turtles and trout, and a sprinkler was always available to jump through.

My first road trip to California showed me a different landscape. Three days' drive from the humid East Coast had me gazing at the Colorado Plateau—the breathtaking canyonlands of the American West, which include parts of Colorado, Utah, Ari-

The Water Gap

- In one year the average American family flushes 8,760 gallons down their low-flow toilets, 29,000 if they're using outdated commodes.

- Each day the average American uses 80 to 100 gallons of water.

- One billion people in the world don't have access to potable water.

- Nearly two billion people don't have adequate sanitation.

- Three million people die each year as a result of preventable water-related diseases.

zona, and New Mexico—which averages less than twelve inches of rainfall a year. This was the real West, with big sky and seemingly infinite miles of open space. Everywhere there was evidence of water realities clashing with cultural fantasies—dams, aquifers, drilling, and pumping—all reaching toward the American belief that "the rain will follow the plow."

I settled in Santa Cruz, California, where there is plenty of water for surfing but little for drinking. Tap water mainly originates from Loch Lomond Reservoir and the San Lorenzo River, which are limited and climate-dependent. The California coast doesn't look like the arid desert of New Mexico, but the facts tell a different story. I've had to learn a few tricks to respect my priv-

Only a Small Fraction of the Water on Earth Is Available for Human Use

- Over 97.5 percent of water on the surface of the Earth is seawater.

- Another 2 percent is in the form of ice such as glaciers and ice caps.

- About 0.5 percent is fresh water, most of which is groundwater, with lake and river water comprising just 0.03 percent.

ilege of living in this climate. Some of these strategies have become a lifestyle and are equally fitting when I return to Connecticut to visit family. Water scarcity is one of the major issues we will have to resolve in the very near future.

WHAT YOU CAN DO
ABOUT HOME ENERGY USE

You can reduce your fuel consumption drastically without buying a single thing by making sure your home and its electrical residents do their job.

Switch your electricity supply to "green power." Every utility assembles a different mix of energy sources. They may generate power by burning their own coal, natural gas, and oil, then supplement that by buying nuclear or water power from other facilities. All five of these sources have serious environmental repercussions; even water power requires huge hydroelectric dams that alter the ecosystem where they are located. Overall, coal is the biggest culprit: 50 percent of all U.S. electricity comes from this greasy black rock. Natural gas—less harmful to the environment but still no angel—supplies 61 percent of home heating.

In sixteen states and the District of Columbia, the power industry has been "restructured" to allow consumers to switch power companies the way they now switch long-distance phone companies. The program is still in its infancy, but as of 2001, 40 percent of American households were able to access renewable power from solar, wind, and hydroelectric sources. In states where power utilities still hold a monopoly, customers can choose a "green pricing" option (e.g., for a slightly higher rate, you can buy green electricity from your longtime

Look for the Green *e*

The Green-e Program (www.green-e.org) awards its logo to forms of electricity it deems "environmentally preferable." The electricity must be derived at least 50 percent from eligible renewable power, have lower air emissions than traditional power, and contain no direct purchases of nuclear power. Look for the logo in any power-company mailings you may receive.

power utility). If green power is available in your area, this is the quickest thing you can do to help the environment. One phone call—to your current company or the green provider in your area—requesting a switch will vastly improve the air everyone breathes. To learn about options in your state, call your power company, visit Green-e (www.green-e.org), or see the Department of Energy's Green Power Network (www.eren.doe.gov/greenpower).

States Allowing Green-Power Competition

As this book goes to press, about fifteen green-power companies are beginning to market their services to customers in these states. If you do not live in one of them, check with the utility that holds a monopoly in your area to see if it offers a "green pricing" option.

Arizona	Massachusetts	Pennsylvania
Connecticut	Michigan	Rhode Island
Delaware	New Hampshire	Texas
Illinois	New Jersey	Virginia
Maine	New York	District of Columbia
Maryland	Ohio	

NOTE: As this book goes to press, green-power legislation is pending in Arkansas, Montana, Nevada, New Mexico, Oklahoma, and Oregon. California, the first state to restructure, has temporarily suspended competition marketing.

Hit the miser switch. All major appliances—fridges, dishwashers, clothes dryers, et cetera—have energy-saver switches. You can still expect essential services from the machines; they will simply do their tasks on the cheap. Fridges, for example, are designed to eliminate condensation in humid weather, which may be unnecessary for your home. A fridge in energy-saver mode shuts off the coils that combat condensation. The energy savers on VCRs shut the machine off after two hours of inactivity; intrepid souls who are not intimidated by their VCRs can program them to turn off after as little as fifteen minutes.

Switch all the bulbs in your home to compact fluorescents.
Once difficult to find, these oddly shaped lightbulbs are now ubiquitous at home centers and hardware stores in a wide array of shapes and wattages. Compact fluorescents (CFLs) burn cooler, last ten times longer, and use 75 percent less energy than Edison's incandescents. Don't let the high cost of CFLs dissuade you from switching. A typical 18-watt bulb (which throws off as much light as a 75-watt incandescent) costs about ten dollars but lasts ten thousand hours; a 75-watt incandescent costs about fifty cents but lasts one thousand hours. So for an extra five bucks you can buy a single CFL that could last seven years, replace ten conventional bulbs, and shave three quarters off your lighting bill. (One maker calculates a total lifetime savings of forty-five dollars per bulb!) If you don't care for the light quality of CFLs, consider natural-spectrum bulbs, which mimic sunlight and last thirty-five hundred hours. Dimmable CFL fixtures can help you save even more electricity. When CFLs do burn out, be sure to recycle them with the rest of your hazardous waste; they contain trace amounts of mercury. (See page 44.)

(See page 44.)

Beware the Torchiere

If you use halogen torchieres, switch immediately to a CFL alternative. Those searingly hot 300- or 500-watt halogen lamps have been implicated in more than one hundred fires and ten deaths nationwide. You will need to buy an entirely new torchiere, since the halogen ones cannot accommodate CFL bulbs.

Switch to rechargeable batteries for small appliances. Flashlights, children's toys, and small electronics such as Walkmans and boom boxes consume a seemingly endless supply of costly batteries. Alkaline and dry batteries release poisonous mercury, cadmium, manganese, and nickel oxides into the environment. Rechargeable nickel metal hydride (NiMH) batteries are nontoxic, can be charged hundreds of times, and work just as well as conventional batteries. Consider switching all your household clocks—including your bedside clock radio—to battery power. They'll never be affected by power outages, and you'll still be rudely awakened in time for work.

Who Else Has Switched to Green Power?

This abbreviated who's who of major companies, schools, cities, towns, and other entities that have switched to green power contains a few surprises.

Birkenstock Footprint Sandals

Carnegie Mellon University

City of Chicago

City of Chula Vista, California

City of Los Angeles

City of Oakland, California

City of Santa Barbara, California

City of Santa Monica, California

City of Seattle

City of Westport, Connecticut

Connecticut College

Fetzer Vineyards

Kinko's

New Belgium Brewing Company, Inc.

Oak Ridge National Laboratory

Patagonia

Penn State University

Sandia National Laboratories

State of Maryland

State of New Jersey

State of New York

U.S. Department of Energy

U.S. Environmental Protection Agency

U.S. Postal Service

TerraPax

Timberland Company

Toyota

Uinta Brewing Company

University of Colorado

University of Pennsylvania

Wesleyan University

Switch all outdoor lights to solar. Self-charging solar lights make perfect sense for outdoor security floodlights, garden paths, and patio lighting. They store energy during the day and go on only when needed. Choose security floodlights with motion detectors to conserve your daytime charge. While you're at it, consider replacing your attic fan with a solar model.

Help your heater do its best. Most houses fritter away the air warmed by the heating system. It's like an endless footrace, with you on the sidelines as the cash-strapped sponsor. Heating costs account for two thirds of household energy bills in the North;

cooling is the second-biggest fuel guzzler nationwide and the top expense in the South. Here are a few things you can do to maximize your heater's efficiency.

- Don't neglect the air filters. Manufacturers recommend replacing the cardboard and fiberglass filters in modern heaters every month during the heating season. This rids the system of excess gunk that can clog it. But instead of endlessly buying and discarding $2 disposable filters, buy a single electrostatic air filter, which costs anywhere from $50 to $150. It will last a lifetime and capture 80 to 90 percent of the airborne particles—dust, pollen, mold, and other allergens—your heater sucks in. In comparison, the disposable filters block 12 percent, tops. Switching greatly reduces paper and fiberglass trash, but you must remember to clean the electrostatic one regularly.

- Vacuum vents and registers regularly.

- Close vents in rooms you don't use often. We're all partial to a toasty-warm potty on chilly mornings, but there's no sense heating and cooling bathrooms when you use them so little throughout the day. You can close the vents and keep the doors to these rooms shut so air doesn't migrate into them.

Use your air conditioner sparingly. Before you reach for the dial, consider these time-honored alternatives:

- Open the windows! Warm days in spring and fall hardly call for a blasting AC. Install fine screens to keep the bugs out, then open the windows and enjoy the fresh air.

- Open the other window. It's called cross-ventilation.

- Use your AC only when you're home.

- If you want to come home to a cool house, program your automatic thermostat to turn on the AC a half hour before you arrive.

- Use a fan rather than AC. You'll use one tenth the electricity.

- Pull shades down when you're not using a room during the day—to keep cool.

Refrigerator wisdom. Always on, never sleeping, your fridge consumes the most energy of all your kitchen appliances, up to 15 percent of a home's total energy usage. (It is second only to heating and cooling systems.) To trim costs associated with running the big lug:

- Set the freezer at 0 to 5 degrees Fahrenheit, the fresh-food compartment at 37 to 40 degrees. If your fridge is old, you may need to experiment to find the optimum setting.

- Cover all dishes of food you keep in the fridge. Humidity rising from them makes the machine work harder. (Use glass lids to reduce consumption of foil and plastic wrap.)

- Shut off the automatic ice maker: a plain old ice tray is more efficient.

- Your fridge runs more efficiently when it's full. An easy way to capitalize on this: fill empty milk or juice cartons with water (don't rinse them first), freeze them, and use the melted ice to water your plants. And you can save your veggie-cooking water for stocks and soups.

- Twice a year, when you set your clocks back and forward, pull the fridge away from the wall and carefully clean the gunk that's collected on the coils behind it.

- Make sure the rubber seals around the doors are tight. If you can close the door on a dollar bill and pull it out, call in a pro to replace the seal.

Cooking Tips. When cooking, use the smallest possible appliance to get the job done. A toaster oven or microwave uses less energy than it takes to heat your oven. A pressure cooker and Crock-Pot eliminate long cooking times on a hot range.

- If the pilot light on your range looks yellow, call a serviceperson. An efficient flame burns blue.

- It pays to clean. Tidy range-top burners and reflectors reflect heat where you want it: the bottom of your pot. Burnt crud absorbs heat like a black turtleneck on a summer's day.

- Keep the flame small enough to fit under your cookware. A flame licking over the sides looks cool but wastes energy. If you're using an electric range, try to match the pot bottom to the element's diameter. (A six-inch pan on an eight-inch burner wastes 40 percent of the energy.)

- Heavy-gauge pots and pans resist warping and maintain contact with the entire flame or element.

- Glass and ceramic pans will cook food in ovens using 25 degrees less heat than metal.

- Don't be in a hurry to preheat. Unless you're Julia Child, you're going to take a while to mix cookie batter or stuff the turkey. Do the work, then preheat. If your oven doesn't have a feature that tells you how hot its interior really is, use a store-bought oven thermometer.

- Open the oven door only when necessary. Oven temps drop 25 degrees every time you open the door.

Clothes drying savvy. Clothes dryers gobble up 10 percent of the energy used in the United States.

- If you can, hang your clothes on a line outdoors. In inclement weather, a line strung up in the basement will do nicely, or wooden clothes-drying racks. I've seen these rigged with cords and pulleys to be lifted toward the ceiling. In small apartments this gets your laundry out of the way and to the hottest part of the room.

- Clean the lint trap before each use of your dryer.

- Dry full loads, not small ones. But don't overstuff the machine.

- You'll save energy and your clothes will last longer if they are not heated to volcanic temperatures in your dryer. Newer dryers come equipped with a moisture sensor. Use it. The machine will shut off when it no longer detects humidity in your clothing.

- Check the outdoor vent occasionally to be sure it's closed when not in use. An open vent is an invitation to outside air—not to mention furry critters.

- While you're at it, go nuts. Clean the excess lint in the vent hood.

- Hang and fold your clothes as soon as they're dry.

IF YOU WANT TO DO MORE

Seal your envelope. This is not a popular pickup line used by heating and cooling professionals. It refers to renovations that ensure not a drop of precious heat in winter or cool air in summer is wasted. Many of these chores are easy enough for homeowners to do themselves.

1. Check and replace the rubber weather stripping around doors and windows. (Rubber weakens over time and no longer forms a tight seal. Ask for "v-seal" weather stripping at the store.)
2. Install door sweeps to keep air from escaping under doors.
3. Rope-caulk drafty windows each winter. This soft putty comes in a roll and can be squeezed into all the nooks and crannies around a window. Once it's in place, you won't be able to open the window until springtime. Save the caulk; it lasts virtually forever and can be used next year. How do you know when to caulk? If your windows are closed and your curtains flutter in the dead of winter, you have either a draft or a poltergeist.
4. Squeegee "low-e" film onto your windows. During the sum-

mer, plastic low-emissivity film keeps solar heat out but lets light in. In winter it stops heat from escaping through the glass. It's affordable—less than a dollar per square foot—and lasts up to ten years. The only downside: it's about as much fun to install as it is to get all the wrinkles out of a used sheet of aluminum foil.

5. Install cellular window blinds. The honeycomb-shaped "cells" in these fabric blinds trap warm air and keep it from migrating to cooler territory. This works in winter and summer. Choose the thickest blinds—the more cells, the more efficient they are.

6. Caulk interior and exterior gaps. You'd be surprised where air escapes. The gaps around electric outlets. Gaps where electric cables, phone lines, and plumbing pipes go from floor to floor or room to room. Gaps where interior walls open up to your attic and basement. You'll find gaps outdoors too, where power and utility lines enter your home, or where your chimney meets the roof. Use 100 percent silicone sealants. They last longest and contain no harmful compounds.

7. Insulate everything: your attic, basement, and walls. The walls are the toughest; you'll need to hire contractors to blow cellulose (a natural substance) through holes in the walls. When buying insulation, choose the highest-rated insulators acceptable for your area. Insulation is identified, labeled, and sold by its resistance to heat flow. The higher its "R-value," the greater the insulating value. The North American Insulation Manufacturers Association website (www.simplyinsulate.com) tells you which R-values are appropriate for your state, calculates your energy savings, and searches for rebates in your area. You can even download how-to videos from the site.

8. Install new windows. Unless you have a new home, you've missed out on the new technology: double-paned windows, argon or krypton gas to block heat, low-e glazing. Today's superwindows boast superior insulating properties—and cost a bundle too. The good news: if you have older double-paned windows, it's more cost-effective to caulk, weather-strip, and install low-e film and cellular shades than it is to replace the old

panes. The best windows have high R-values and low U-values (low level of heat transfer) and are certified by the National Fenestration Rating Council. Two websites (www.efficient windows.org and www.nfrc.org) teach the basics and give tips for understanding NFRC labels.

Install an automatic thermostat on your heater. In older homes and apartments with manual thermostats, it's easy to forget to turn down the heat at night. An automatic thermostat can be programmed once per season and left to do its job. Set it to correspond to your family's daily rhythms: lower nighttime temps in winter when you're under the covers, warmer daytime temps in summer when no one's home, et cetera. If the weather changes dramatically, you can always adjust it. By turning your thermostat back 10 or 15 degrees for eight hours, you can save 5 to 15 percent a year on your heating bill.

Replace the gasket (or "rubber weather stripping") inside your oven door. This gasket locks heat in but deteriorates with age and heat. Check that it's still supple and forms a tight seal. If not, replace it.

Plant "energy trees." In the northern states plant deciduous trees on the south and west sides of your house. They'll shade your abode in summer and let sunlight warm you in winter after leaves have fallen. Evergreens planted on the north side shield homes from harsh winter wind. In southern regions, evergreens to the south and west of your home offer shade year-round. Properly placed trees and shrubs can reduce heating and cooling costs a whopping 25 percent—unless you start running power to the tree house. Note: large trees should never be planted closer than 30 feet from the foundation of your home. Before you plant, seek the advice of a landscaper or arborist.

Buying Energy-Efficient Appliances

One way to judge the efficiency of a big appliance is to read its yellow-and-black Energy Guide label. Federal law requires these stickers on most large appliances. An arrow on the scale shows how the item you're considering compares with other models in terms of efficiency. You'll even learn the model's estimated annual cost. But you won't learn which competing products do better. For that information, check back issues of *Consumer Reports* or the website and publications of the American Council for an Energy-Efficient Economy (www.aceee.org).

In 1992 the EPA (and later the Department of Energy) introduced a voluntary labeling program called Energy Star (www.energystar.gov) to identify products that are especially energy-efficient. To qualify for an Energy Star, the product must *exceed* the federally mandated efficiency standard in its appliance category. Do Energy Star products cost more? Yes and no. Computers have always been remarkably efficient, and Energy Star status does not affect their cost. You will notice a price difference in the big stuff discussed below. But by paying up front for a better machine, you save on energy (and water) for the rest of the product's life span. You may even be eligible for a rebate from the manufacturer, your utility company, or your town—sometimes all three!

Heaters. To qualify for Energy Star status, furnaces must demonstrate a 90 percent "annual fuel utilization efficiency" (AFUE); boilers, 85 percent AFUE. Air-source heat pumps must meet a minimum "seasonal energy-efficiency rating" (SEER) of 12 and a "heating season performance factor" (HSPF) of 7.6. Geosource heat pumps should have a minimum "energy-efficiency rating" (EER) of 14.1 and a minimum "coefficient of performance" (COP) of 3.3.

Air conditioners. Resist the temptation to buy more power than you need. A bigger room AC doesn't get rid of hot, humid air quicker. It leaves you with a roomful of damp, muggy air. Carefully measure the room. If you're installing a central system, ask the installer not to stop at measuring the rooms in your house but to inspect the level and quality of your insulation. Energy Star central ACs must meet a minimum SEER of 12. Room ACs must meet the minimum EER shown on the chart.

ROOM ACS

SIZE	EER
Less than 6,000 btu	10.7
6,000–7,999 btu	10.7
8,000–13,999 btu	10.8
14,000–19,999 btu	10.7
20,000 btu or greater	9.4

Ranges/ovens. Gas appliances use much less energy than their electric cousins. Every chef worth his toque touts gas ranges, which let you use only as much heat as you need and no more. Models with an electric-pilot ignition save even more. If you need to use electric, know that halogen and induction elements use less energy than those old electric coils. The catch: you can't use aluminum cookware. Consider buying a self-cleaning oven. They use less energy because they're better insulated, although running the cycle more than once a month might eat up the gains. (This is the one time it pays to be a slob.) Cleaning after baking, when the oven is still hot, saves energy.

Clothes dryers. When buying, remember gas dryers use less energy than electric: twenty cents a load compared with forty cents.

Refrigerators. Skip the fancy gadgets: ice makers, water dispensers, butter churners, and shoe buffers. They represent greater profit to the salesperson but diminish the machine's efficiency. Freezer-on-top models are the most efficient style. Make sure the old fridge is recycled responsibly. (Most important, you want to

Hope for Greener Cooling

Even if you're conscientious about buying energy-efficient air conditioners and refrigerators, they will still assault the environment in an insidious way that is different from other appliances. The foam insulation in U.S. fridges contains chemicals called hydrochlorofluorocarbons (HCFCs), which are known to damage the ozone layer. And the refrigerants in these appliances, HFCs (hydrofluorocarbons), are among the most potent greenhouse gases ever invented. Manufacturers shifted to these chemicals when even worse ozone-killers, chlorofluorocarbons (CFCs), were targeted for a worldwide ban in 1987. (These notorious gases continue to leak from old refrigerants, spray cans, Styrofoam cups, food trays, and packaging.) The new gases are not due to be phased out until 2030—a date some say is too far off. Environmentalists hound corporations to eliminate HCFCs and HFCs from their appliances, but industry has been reluctant, saying it would be too costly to switch to natural refrigerants at once. Think of all the food warehouses that would need to be retrofitted! Meanwhile, all of these refrigerants continue to be traded on international black markets, since prices have been rising and it's often hard to recharge old appliances.

Natural solutions do exist. In Europe, Whirlpool and others use a technology called Greenfreeze, in which cooling is performed by small amounts of natural gases such as propane or isobutane. Until all chlorine-based chemicals are eliminated from appliances, consumers can:

- Live without refrigerators or AC.

- Move to Europe.

- Use these appliances responsibly.

- Investigate "green" cooling and refrigerating options. A California company called Sun Frost sells refrigerators whose refrigerants are chlorine-free (but the insulating foam does contain these chemicals). The fridges run on a mere half kilowatt-hour per day. (If you have an old fridge, chances are you're burning about five kilowatt-hours a day!)

make sure the refrigerant and foam insulation are recycled.) Most department stores and white-goods sellers participate in recycling programs. If you're unsure what happens to your old fridge, ask. *Don't* move the old one into the garage to chill your brewskis. You have a nice thing going here. Why blow it?

What You Can Do About Water

Shower smarter. If taking a shower is your primary mental-health pleasure, enjoy it. Showers can be more efficient than baths. Consider taking shorter showers or installing an efficient showerhead, especially if you are in the habit of showering more than once a day. Try wetting, lathering with the water turned off, then rinsing.

Don't let the water run. Many of us not only let the water run when brushing our teeth, washing our hands, or doing dishes, but we let it run full force. Turn it off and turn it down. Also, cleaning is more effective when you don't dilute the cleanser.

Switch to earth-friendly soaps, shampoos, and detergents. Soap—the natural result of chemical reaction between fats and bases—has been around for centuries and has always been biodegradable. Unfortunately, many bar "soaps" sold today are actually detergents in brick form. Detergents are another story. They often contain phosphates to disperse stains and dislodge food particles. Phosphorus dumped into the water supply can easily overwhelm the environment. (Overfertilized by phosphates, algae invades waterways and dies, robbing other plant and animal life of precious oxygen.) You can mitigate the damage by switching to gentler, plant-based liquid and bar soaps. Plant-based soaps are made with vegetable oils, cocoa butter, baking soda, hydrogen peroxide, citric acid, vinegar, and herbal extracts and are biodegradable. The primary fat in ultramild castile soaps, for example, is olive oil. You can also look for phosphate-free detergents and dishwasher soaps. (Dishwashing liquids are usually phosphate-free.) If you keep the water pure, you'll feel better about reusing it to water your plants during a drought. And if it's just going down the drain, you won't be contributing to ground-water contamination. If you drop off your laundry to be done at a Laundromat, bring them your preferred detergent.

Use your washing machine more efficiently.

- Most of us overwash our clothes. Wearing a shirt or a pair of jeans once does not necessarily mean it needs to be tossed in the hamper.

- Full loads are more efficient to wash than partial loads.

- Avoid hot-water settings. Your clothes will still get clean when washed in cold or warm water and in less detergent. Experiment to see which mix works best for you.

- Try using half the detergent recommended by the manufacturer.

Be dishwasher-savvy.

- It's more efficient to use the dishwasher than to wash dishes, glasses, and cutlery by hand—but only if you do full loads.

- Use the energy-saver feature on your dishwasher. It takes a little longer to dry the dishes, but so what? Dry is dry.

- Wash big pots and pans by hand. Getting them out of the way allows you to fit more stuff in the dishwasher.

Lower your water temperature. Water heaters are energy hogs; you can save watts of energy and wads of cash by lowering the thermostat to 120 degrees Fahrenheit. This is more than sufficient for most homes. (Each 10-degree reduction saves you about 5 percent in heating costs.) If you have small kids, this also ensures that they don't scald themselves. And when you go on vacation, lower the temperature as much as possible or shut the heater

The Deal with Drinking Water

If you and your family currently buy jugs or single-serving containers of bottled water, it may surprise you to learn that the water in the bottles doesn't always hail from the pristine sylvan locales depicted on the label. The only way to know what's in the bottle is to read the fine print. New FDA regulations recognize nine different types of water—artesian, fluoridated, ground, mineral, purified, sparkling, spring, sterile, and well water—and bottlers are required to use one of these terms on the label to identify their product. Municipal water is the source of 25 percent of the bottled water sold in the United States. Once this water is processed, it can be sold as "purified" water—at 240 to 10,000 times the price!

In a four-year study conducted by the Natural Resources Defense Council, scientists found in some bottled water the same contaminants found in municipal water: bacteria, industrial solvents, chemicals from plastic, and even arsenic. When you factor in that plastic water bottles never biodegrade, and that the best recycling efforts have never kept up with the multitudes of plastic bottles, it makes sense to look for alternatives to store-bought water. One choice is to contract a water-cooler service that supplies water in reusable glass bottles. If you want to eliminate even the fuel used to transport these, you might consider a home purification system. This opens another can of worms. Or, shall we say, bottle of water. Systems differ in quality and the types of impurities they weed out. So before you spend a dime, it pays to know what's in your water. It makes no sense to buy a two-thousand-dollar distiller system when a twenty-dollar pitcher will strain out what little contaminants are found in your water.

Request a copy of your water utility's annual water-quality (or "consumer confidence") report. This reveals impurities typically found in your community's water. If you are still concerned, you might want to have your tap water privately tested. Armed with these two pieces of data, you can then visit the website of NSF International (www.nsf.org), a nonprofit public-safety corporation that certifies water-purification systems. Their search engine (www.nsf.org/Certified/DWTU) lets you select contaminants you need to eliminate and tells you which systems might fit your needs.

off altogether. Just be sure you know how to turn it back on, or light the pilot light if it's a gas model.

IF YOU WANT TO DO MORE

Invest in water-saving hardware. Faucet aerators and low-flow showerheads, available in hardware stores for under twenty dollars, restrict the amount of water coming out of taps without sacrificing pressure. (Federal standards now require new showerheads to operate at 2.5 gallons per minute and new aerators at .5 to 1 gpm—but you may be able to find ones that are slightly more efficient.) Choose lever showerheads that let you shut off the water when you're lathering up.

Save water with every flush. A plastic toilet dam inserted into an old tank holds back as much as one or two gallons of water per flush. You can achieve the same result by inserting a two-liter plastic soda bottle or a one-gallon water bottle—weighted with pebbles and filled with water—into the tank. The most efficient option: upgrading to a low-flow toilet. Older toilets waste as much as 7 gallons per flush, while new ones use only 1.6 gallons.

Buy an insulating jacket for your water heater. This is one of the top ten do-it-yourself projects: for twenty bucks you shave 9 percent off your heating costs. Be sure to insulate the top of the tank and the first ten feet of the pipe carrying the hot water out.

Garden smart. Plant drought-resistant plants, which require less water to live. (We'll tell you more about this technique, called xeriscaping, in chapter 9.) Use drip hoses and low-flow nozzles and sprinklers. Install timers that let you water your garden for a specific period of time, then shut off.

Capture rainwater. Water from the sky is just the thing for outdoor jobs like watering plants, washing your car, and scrubbing down the patio or pooch. Buy a rain barrel from a gardener's supply company. You can even splurge and get a nifty attachable hose for linking up two barrels.

Repairing and Replacing
Your Water-Loving Appliances

However durable, washing machines, dishwashers, and hot-water heaters inevitably need to be replaced, setting off a chain reaction of acquisition and disposal. When you buy a spanking new machine, the old one ends up on the trash heap, along with all the packing material. Fortunately, you wield enormous power during these transactions. First, consider repairing the appliance. There is something to be said for keeping your machine out of the waste stream in the first place. If that's not feasible, replace it with a model that is more efficient. In general, gas appliances use less energy than electric ones. And appliances built before 1990 will not incorporate newer federal-efficiency standards. See the discussion on Energy Guide labels and Energy Star products on page 61.

Before you buy, grill the salespeople. Most department stores now participate in recycling programs. Be specific. Ask them what will happen to the machine they take back from you. Appliances like refrigerators and air conditioners contain hydrochlorofluorocarbons (HCFCs), chemical compounds known to damage the ozone layer. Will that material be recovered? Also ask if they will recycle the white foam blocks (expanded polystyrene, or PS #6) your new product will no doubt come packaged in.

Or consider donating your old machine. Charities such as the Salvation Army or Goodwill may accept it. Other organizations—schools, houses of worship, senior centers, and hospitals—may need desperately what you're tossing out, and have volunteer handymen in the wings waiting to repair it.

When your new appliance is delivered, take responsibility for the resulting trash. Sort and recycle the cardboard and plastic. You might also ask local packing and shipping franchises (such as

Mailboxes Etc. or Pak Mail) if they will accept the foam blocks. As a last resort, check the website of the Alliance of Foam Packaging Recyclers (www.epspackaging.org) for a drop-off site or mail-in address near you.

Washing machines. The average household washes four hundred full loads of laundry a year, using 40 gallons of water a load with a conventional washer. In comparison, an Energy Star–rated washer uses only 18 to 25 gallons per load. Savings: 7,000 gallons of water a year, not to mention the energy needed to run the machine and heat the water. How do they do it? Special sensors judge how full the washer is and adjust the water accordingly. The front-loading tub spins faster and longer, squeezing out more water so your clothes need less drying.

10 Things to Do Instead of Showering a Second or Third Time Today

1. Pretend you're starring in your very own reality TV show.
2. Really get to know the next telemarketer who calls up.
3. Barter a peace agreement between your cat and dog.
4. Repopularize the Macarena.
5. Become a movie star; start salad-dressing and spaghetti-sauce company.
6. Learn the way to San Jose.
7. Count the Starbucks in your neighborhood. Wait ten minutes. Count them again.
8. Build an addition to your Barbie Dream House.
9. Sit around with a smug look on your face.
10. Stand outside with a bar of soap and pray for rain.

Dishwashers. Water in a dishwasher must be at least 140 degrees Fahrenheit to clean dishes. That's one reason plumbers set hot-water heaters at 150 degrees Fahrenheit. Newer dishwashers heat their own water, so you can save 10 percent in heating costs by lowering the water-heater thermostat to 120 degrees.

ENERGY
AND WATER

69

Water heaters. The most common type of water heater features a giant storage tank in which the water is kept hot and toasty for your eventual use. There's the rub: you're heating water you don't necessarily need at that moment. And when heat escapes through the walls of the tank, the heater fires up again to keep the water at the minimum temperature. Water heaters are the biggest energy consumers in your home, after the heating and cooling systems.

Consider buying a tankless ("on-demand") water heater. Popular in Europe, these models heat water only as it is used, so you're not paying to heat and keep a huge tank of hot water on standby. Smaller units do have some limitations—they can run only one or two large appliances or fixtures at a time. But a reputable installer will be able to correctly size the system to the home.

ONE LAST WORD . . . TAKE A GREEN TOUR

Walk through every room in your home and take a hard look at your appliances. If you're like most people, your outlets are a life-support system for toasters, blenders, food processors, TVs, VCRs, stereos, DVD players, computers, printers, lamps, power tools, and seldom-used hand vacuums.

- Ask yourself how often you use these things. Do your possessions really fit your needs and interests? Do you have a food processor because it once seemed like a good idea? Does your bedroom TV go unused because you really like to read before bed? Consider donating your superfluous appliances to charitable organizations, hospitals, and local senior centers. Each donated item means one does not have to be bought and driven home, and its packaging tossed out.

- Decide what really matters to you and your family. If quiet time together is hard to come by, challenge everyone to wean themselves off TV one night a week, then two, then three . . .

- If you need to replace even the tiniest appliance, choose an energy-efficient one. Believe it or not, there are Energy Star answering machines. Or choose small appliances that will run on rechargeable batteries.

- When not using an appliance, unplug it. Plug several appliances into a power strip with an on-off switch. Use that switch.

- You may, understandably, choose to leave some appliances—answering machines, clocks, VCRs—on continuously to keep set preferences. For some, that's not a priority. One of our friends says his VCR flashes "12:00" all the time. He doesn't care because he's covered it with a piece of electrician's tape. And even a broken clock tells the correct time twice a day.

CHAPTER 4

COMMUNICATION

What we have here is a failure to communicate.
—Cool Hand Luke

While I was growing up, my family moved between California and Connecticut millions of times—or so it seemed to me. At each new home I could count on finding a newspaper at the door every morning. It was a simple but comforting fact that no matter where I lived I would always have a sufficient amount of lining material for my birdcages.

This made an impression on me, and today I know the location of every vendor in Santa Cruz County that sells *The New York Times.* My father is happy to note that I'm now reading the paper before turning it into a litter box.

These days I start my morning with a freshly laid egg from a chicken in the backyard, a thick slice of sourdough toast, NPR, and *The New York Times.* It's my way of keeping my connection to the world. Unless, of course, the surf is up. Then I skip the paper and grab the surfboard.

Communicating and staying connected with the rest of the world do carry what environmentalists call a "resource price"— and my habits are no exception. Printing the national Sunday edition of *The New York Times,* for example, uses seventy-five thousand trees. I also read *The Nation,* which, since it's a small weekly magazine (small publication, big ideas), is easier to negotiate after returning home from a few weeks of travel. I should probably kick both these habits, since both publications are available online, for free (www.nytimes.com and www.thenation.com).

For the time being, I'll keep my daily paper, but I'd like to share some ideas about how to be a powerful activist while staying in touch with family, community, and friends, and keeping up with what's going on in the world.

YACKETYYACKYACKYACK

A letter came in the mail one day for the president of Working Assets, an unusual phone company that gives 1 percent of its revenues each year to progressive nonprofit organizations. Enclosed in the envelope was a photo of a horse, and to phrase it delicately, I'm not talking about the front of the horse. The note was from one of Working Assets' 370,000 customers, who disagreed with the company's stance on gun control. "Dear Sir," the letter began, "You are a horse's ass, and I'd like you to know that . . ."

The letter still hangs in the company's San Francisco offices, and not only because it made everyone laugh. If there's one thing Michael Kieschnick, the company's president and cofounder, has learned about his customers in fifteen years of business, it's that they're passionately addicted to giving the company a piece of their mind.

"Our customers are educated and like to talk to us," Michael says. "They send us letters and e-mails with suggestions for other groups we should give money to. They tell us what political issues we should take on. Authors who've written books on these topics send us their books. They're pretty active customers."

Michael's proud of that, and even a little surprised. He's the first to admit that Working Assets is not exactly the world's most glamorous business. The company buys access to phone networks in bulk and sells it to its customers. Nothing fancy there. The things that separate the company from other long-distance carriers are the spirit of the customers and what Working Assets does with its revenues.

The company is one of a growing number that have managed to turn rather dull consumer products into forces for social and environmental change. These days consumers everywhere are shelling out monthly fees for phone service, cell phones, Internet providers, pocket e-mail devices, and heaven knows what else. Now there's a way to make sure that some of that money goes to people and causes that really need it.

If the idea sounds odd to you, join the club. When Michael and his partners, Peter Barnes and Laura Scher, began Working Assets in 1985, their product was not phone service but credit cards. The trio argued endlessly about the irony inherent to their business model. Was it right to encourage people to spend their way to a better planet? "We wouldn't have that argument today," Michael says. "If you're going to buy something, why not buy in a way that helps?"

In 1986, the company gave away thirty-two thousand dollars to sixteen groups. By 2001, the number had climbed to six million—one million of that generated by customers voluntarily "rounding up" when they pay their phone bill. (The extra cash goes right into the donations pool.) "Those nickels and dimes add up quickly," Michael explains.

Of course, since the company shares its revenues with more than fifty organizations, customers occasionally will disagree with their choices and politics. The guy who sent that horse picture to Michael sure did.

But get this: he's still a customer.

TOWARD A GREENER WEB

The country's first major "green" Internet company, EcoISP, was started by a guy who got his start selling dirt. The year was 1961, and Paul Gerstenberger was only four years old. His dad was a young college student, his mom a waitress who baby-sat on the side. Mom, Dad, Paul, and his brother and sister were all living in a housing project in Seattle.

One morning Paul's mom came downstairs to find someone had broken into their home and stolen her purse. She had only twelve dollars in it, but that money was supposed to last her a whole week. You had to be darn frugal to make twelve dollars last that long, even in 1961. Mrs. G. watched every dime, but now she didn't know what she was going to do.

Watching her, Paul was seized with two powerful feelings: compassion for his mother, who was hurting bad, and determination to do something to make her feel better.

A few days later, he was playing outside when he saw a neighbor dump some potting soil from a plastic bag onto her houseplants. Paul thought that was the weirdest thing: dirt from a plastic bag. Later, after the neighbor had gone, he plucked the bag out of the trash and saw it had a price tag on it: ten cents. *Shoot,* he thought, *I can do better than this.*

And he did. A few days later he was selling dirt door-to-door. Ten cents a bucket. Pretty soon Paul was hiring other kids to help him dig and sift.

That was the beginning of Paul's career as an entrepreneur. He also sold blackberries, hired himself out to mow lawns, clean garages, or sweep dog poop off people's properties. He passed along his earnings to his mom, who repaid him with a hug. Okay, sometimes he bought himself a string of licorice too.

In October 2001 Paul went into the media business. He and some partners launched a grass-roots alternative to the big Internet-service providers. A customer can log on for less than the big providers charge, and Paul donates 50 percent of his profits to each customer's favorite environmental group.

"Everything I do these days," he says, "is trying to help solve a really big problem and make a few bucks on the side. With this venture, I wanted to figure out a way to give environmental groups enough power and money to keep on fighting."

People doubted it would work. The business and trade magazines all asked how a tiny website could take on the likes of AOL or Yahoo, which constantly bombard Americans with TV advertising. Paul knew, though, that environmental groups had something these other businesses could only dream of: passionate, committed members. Paul phoned every environmental group he could think of and asked them to do him a favor: would they mind mentioning or sending his website's CD in their next mailing? If customers signed up, he said, they would probably choose to donate their fee to the very organization that had made the CD available.

He was right. He is on target to reach his one-million-customer goal by December 2003.

That ain't dirt.

Paper Doesn't Grow on Trees

The book you're reading is printed on paper that all of us helped produce. It's made entirely from "postconsumer" waste. You might think this is no big deal, but it is. "100 percent recycled" is a misleading term. Only "100 percent postconsumer content" guarantees that no trees were cut in the making of that paper.

Here's why. Paper mills are allowed to call scrap fiber lying around their factories "recycled"—even though it has never left the premises. Most recycled paper is 70 percent unused virgin fiber scraps and 30 percent postconsumer. While it's certainly good to reuse the scraps, it's even better to give a second and even third life to previously used paper. And as more and more of us do this, 100 percent postconsumer paper will become cheaper to make and easier to find.

We told our publisher we wanted the real deal. That took some doing: 100 percent postconsumer paper is pricier, and few manufacturers carry it. (It's hard to find in retail stores too, but we'll show you where to order it online.) After some sleuthing, our publisher found Jeff Mendelsohn, a thirty-five-year-old recycled-paper king.

Jeff's a guy after our own hearts. Growing up amid San Diego's beaches and deserts, he cultivated what he calls "a deep personal appreciation for nature." His San Francisco–based company, New Leaf, is trying to reverse a century-old tradition of negatively impacting the environment to make paper. For a long time, the big companies didn't think there was a real market for recycled paper. De-inking and repulping adds to the cost, and manufacturers have long observed that Americans do a better job of recycling paper than they do of buying it back.

Jeff and a few other pioneers are laying a different bet. They think once consumers know there's a better product out there, the market will grow. To make the paper environmentally committed folks want, they needed to hire a paper mill to make some samples. At the first industry convention Jeff attended in 1993, he couldn't get a single appointment. "We got laughed at in the beginning," he recalls. "It was hard to get the attention of the major mills."

But that's changing. Today, all the Harry Potter books in Canada are printed on New Leaf's paper. And all Kinko's stores carry the company's copier paper; consumers simply need to ask for it.

Start reading the labels the next time you're buying stationery or printer and copier paper. "High postconsumer content of more than, say, thirty to forty percent is the first thing to look for," Jeff says. "*Recycled* is a rather meaningless term without an indication of what percent is postconsumer."

- One ton (forty cartons) of 30 percent postconsumer-content copier paper saves 7.2 trees.

- One ton of 50 percent post-consumer-content copier paper saves 12 trees.

(*Source: Conservatree*)

WHAT YOU CAN DO

Here are some ways you can be a force for change even when you're just staying in touch with loved ones or keeping up with what's going on in the world.

The Telephone

Do you screen your calls? I'm not answering that question, but if it were not for my phone machine, I'd have to talk to phone companies every evening about rates, minutes, and plans. All these choices seem about as inspiring as shopping for picture hooks. Thankfully, there is an opportunity here for some effective armchair activism.

Read on and you'll find some good news if you use a cell phone too. (I'm not personally afraid of electromagnetic radiation. I hold a cell phone to my head for half an hour per day.) Some developing countries have skipped the entire conventional phone system and have gone wireless. Imagine: cell phones in the rice fields of Mongolia. That's global communication with less impact on resources.

> *There are fewer phone lines in the entire continent of Africa than there are in either Manhattan or Tokyo.*
> *—Dr. Yvonne Muthien*

Make the switch to a socially responsible carrier.

- Working Assets (www.workingassets.com) offers telephone long distance, cellular phones, and credit cards. Their current promotion is the sweetest deal in town: newcomers receive sixty free minutes for the first six months, and a free pint of any Ben & Jerry's concoction each month for a year. Beyond the sweet creams, as we went to press they were offering four different long-distance options, two types of calling cards, and a very competitive cell-phone package.

- Earth Tones (www.earthtones.com) is a long-distance phone company owned by a consortium of environmental organizations, including state Public Interest Research Groups, the National Environmental Law Center, the Toxics Action Center, Earth Day Resources, Campaign to Save the Environment, and others. Founded in 1993, the company operates like a co-op: buying long-distance access in bulk, then selling it to customers at a savings. Since the green folks own the company, they keep 100 percent of the profits to fund their ongoing work. The key to Earth Tones' savings lies primarily in the way they bill you. Most long-distance companies round calls up to the nearest minute. You'd be billed 4 minutes for a call that lasted exactly 3 minutes, 3 seconds. Earth Tones bills in 6-second increments, so the same call would be billed as 3.1 minutes. Earth Tones says that this practice, along with a dearth of add-on fees and charges, saves customers 5 to 10 percent over traditional plans. Earth Tones offers both business and residential plans. At the time we went to press, they were offering three different long-distance plans, three types of calling cards, and the option to have Earth Tones assume your cellular long-distance coverage and convert your current plan to their flat minute-by-minute fee.

Mounting Tide of Mobiles

Americans are discarding 130 million cell phones each year. Over the next five years, that will amount to sixty-five thousand tons added to landfills. What can you do? Check to see if your mobile carrier has a phone-recycling program. Some organizations, such as Wireless Foundation (www.wirelessfoundation.org), modify phones so they can only dial 911, and distribute them free to neighborhood watches, victims of domestic abuse, or senior citizens. Sprint, for example, already offers drop-off boxes in its stores and presents donors with tax-deductible receipts. If such programs are not available in your area, check with your local recycling program to see if they will accept the phone, the battery, or both.

The Internet

Writer Wendell Berry, one of my heroes, doesn't own a computer. This makes me feel better when mine crashes or I can't get something to print. I think to myself, "I will just grab a pencil and paper. I'll go simple, not supporting the energy companies or computer companies. I'll unplug all my appliances!"

I don't need the EPA or the NRDC website to tell me about the environmental crisis. I can feel it in my bones. But I do find e-mail to be a powerful and efficient tool and the Internet to be extremely educational, if I can keep my search focused and not surf too much. Wendell Berry doesn't surf, so he has no need for the California Surf Report (www.slonet.org/~tsulaiti/surfreport), one of my favorite bookmarks. The Internet is a choice I've added to my life, so I've researched a few methods that keep my conscience clear:

Dial-up access through Denver-based EcoISP (www.ecoisp.com) costs less than AOL's standard fee and provides six e-mail addresses, chat rooms, discussion forums, and a smart website that features environmental news, surveys of important green websites, shopping links, and games.

Let the Web help you eliminate paper use. Write, edit, and deliver paperless documents to far-flung family members by sending e-mail attachments. It's an instant darkroom, too. Digital cameras can help stop the flow of waste from photo-finishing labs. Snap your photos and e-mail them to family members without ever setting foot in a photo-finishing shop.

Print responsibly. It's so cheap and easy to print everything we see online—driving directions, news stories, movie reviews, recipes—that families can easily burn through a case of paper every few months. (One ream—five hundred sheets—uses up 6 percent of a tree!) Ink-jet cartridges are not cheap, but we think nothing of tossing out these ink-besmirched, indestructible plastic containers and popping in new ones. Here are ways you can press back the tide of junk.

- **Print on both sides of every sheet of paper you have.**
- **Use scrap sheets of printer or copier paper for grocery lists and notes.**
- **Recycle all home office paper.** According to the EPA,

Kid Project: A "Clean" Family Tree

Challenge your kids to assemble a family tree showing off photos of everyone—even their most far-flung relatives—with a minimum of waste.

How to do it: To reduce fossil-fuel consumption and packaging waste, ask relatives to e-mail images. Ask your kids to manipulate text and images and preview their work onscreen before printing a single item.

paper in all its forms accounts for 40 percent of all the solid waste generated in the United States—and a quarter of it is white office paper. Sadly, only about 20 percent of the nation's office paper is recycled.

• **Choose recycled paper with the highest postconsumer waste content possible.** (Unbleached, recycled paper is best for your body and the earth.) Hold off buying an entire case until you find a brand and grade of paper you like. If you're ordering paper online, choose vendors closest to you, so your delivery doesn't consume tankers of gasoline just getting to your door. Contact GreenLine Paper in Pennsylvania (www.greenlinepaper.com); GreenCo in Vermont (1-800-326-2897); Treecycle in Montana (www.treecycle .com); and Real Earth Environmental in California (www .treeco.com).

• **Recycle your laser toner cartridges.** Most companies that manufacture laser printers (Apple, Hewlett-Packard, and Canon among them) have excellent recycling programs. Your new cartridge comes with a prepaid shipping label; when the ink runs out, you repack it, affix the label, and either drop it off at the designated carrier or phone for a pickup. It's something to keep in mind when buying a printer or stocking up on cartridges.

• **Refill your own ink cartridges.** A number of stationery-supply companies now sell ink in bulk. Customers buy a "refill kit" that comes with instructions, latex gloves, and an assortment of syringes that make it easy to refill and use your current ink cartridges again and again. The prices are incredible. For the same twenty dollars you spend on a single ink-jet cartridge, you can refill your own ten to fifteen times. You'll never have to toss out an ink-contaminated cartridge again. Suppliers include Mr. Inkjet (www.misterinkjet.com), All-Ink (www.all-ink.com), Inksell (www.inksell.com), and Inkville (www.inkville.com).

> *My mom doesn't let anything go to waste. She tears the pages of movie scripts either she or Dad have rejected into quarters and uses the backs as scrap. Now and then I'll get a note in the mail: "Here's the book you wanted. Love, Mom." On the other side will be fragments of bad movie dialogue: "Let's get outta here!"*

The Price of White

Mother Nature has been bleached out of every scrap of paper in a maddening quest for unadulterated whiteness. What do paper manufacturers use to give us the white paper we crave? Chlorine gas and chlorine dioxide. When chlorine reacts with other materials in the paper-making process, it produces a variety of toxic chemical compounds called dioxins, which can pollute nearby skies and streams. Dioxins have been shown to be carcinogenic, but manufacturers say very little of these chemicals end up in the products we touch. Besides office paper, Americans buy, handle, and consume such bleached-paper products as envelopes, facial tissues, napkins, toilet paper, baby wipes, tampons, coffee filters, and tea bags, just to name a few. If you want to take steps toward a dioxin-free home, choose recycled paper that is "processed chlorine-free" (PCF) or new paper that is "totally chlorine-free" (TCF). These are bleached with hydrogen peroxide, which breaks down into water and air.

Snail Mail

Nothing compares with a handwritten thank-you note or letter received in the mail. You can make everything you write something special if you simply take the time to think before buying stationery supplies.

- Reduce the waste stream by switching to refillable pens instead of using disposables.

- Use recycled-paper stationery.

- Buy self-sticking labels so you can reuse junk-mail envelopes.

- Use blank postcards instead of cards and envelopes. You can even cut the front of greeting cards and use as postcards.

- To reduce junk mail in one fell swoop, go to www.opt-out.cdt.org.

Newspapers and Magazines

You may have noticed that more than 50 percent of any newsstand magazine consists of advertising, except for certain women's magazines, which are 100 percent advertising. Okay, I'm joking, but it wouldn't hurt to reevaluate each subscription as it comes due, and save all that paper.

- Get your news online. Most online newspapers and news networks allow registered users to specify their favorite subjects and to receive customized links to those articles in their e-mailboxes each day.

- If you read a story online that you'd like to keep, resist the impulse to print it out. E-mail a copy of the story to yourself. This allows you to create a paper-free archive of interesting articles whose text you can easily search or forward to friends. It beats photocopying the same article again and again.

What About Alternative Fibers?

Alternative fibers such as hemp, flax, and kenaf are slowly being recognized as perfect ecological substitutes for wood products. Hemp is a distant relative of marijuana, without the psychoactive effects. Kenaf is a pretty flowering plant in the hibiscus family. Flax is the plant that gives us linseed oil and linen and whose nutritious seeds provide necessary essential fatty acids. All three plants have been cultivated for centuries, grow more quickly than trees, and generate vast quantities of usable fiber. Hemp, which is still illegal to grow in most of the United States, produces more pulp per acre than timber, can be recycled more often than wood-pulp fibers, and resists mold and ultraviolet light. While it's a good idea to buy fabrics and clothing made from these products (hemp *products,* including clothing made from imported fabric, are legal in the United States), I still think it makes more sense to buy recycled paper with a high postconsumer-waste content. Using the recycled waste we already have is the surest way to keep trees from being cut down.

Getting Your News Green

The fate of the planet depends on all of us staying informed. But green news is hard to find on conventional online news sites. For example, an energy package that Congress is considering might be found in the politics section. The new plastics-recycling technology might be in sci-tech. A review of hot new solar-power companies might be found in the business section. If you live for this stuff, you might consider getting all your green news in one place. See the Resources Directory for good green news sources.

- Consider sharing magazine subscriptions with a friend or group of friends or colleagues. This works really well if one person can flag interesting articles. After all, few of us have enough time to read all the mags that pile up.

The Case for More Radio . . .

There is a sweetness and simplicity about radio that television has never approached. The simplest radios don't require electric outlets. They don't even need batteries. Once upon a time, kids built radios from scratch, with parts they found around the house or in electronics stores. On summer nights you can still place a wireless radio outdoors and listen to a ballgame while you cook out. Try *that* with TV. (Actually, please don't.) Later, as night falls, you can listen to music and still have a conversation or help the kids with school projects. Radio makes kitchen and home chores go down easy. Listening to the radio frees your eyes for other tasks and engages your imagination too. No matter where you are—even if you're flat on your back in a starlit campsite thousands of miles from home—you can go to bed knowing how your team fared in the big game. Beautiful.

. . . And Less TV

American kids watch twenty-one hours of TV each week, witness thirty-one thousand commercials a year, and as a result learn to crave bad food and a universe of wasteful plastic toys. If you're worried about your family's devotion to the living room Cyclops, you might want to tame the beast. Try to place limits on viewing time. Pick only shows that matter. Videotape your favorite shows and fast-forward through commercials. (Technology such as TiVo may simplify this process in the coming years.) If you have kids, stockpile a library of wonderful videos or DVDs for them to choose from. Now and then, pick a film you loved as a child and watch it with your family as you would a first-run movie.

One Last Word . . .

Until we convert to using tree-free paper, here are a few suggestions for what to do with those printed pages.

You can donate your used books out of the kindness of your heart. Churches, synagogues, senior centers, hospitals, and library-clearance sales may gratefully accept them. You can donate used books for filthy lucre. Thrift shops will take donations in exchange for a tax-deductible receipt. You can post your books on a website such as half.com (www.half.com) and reap, yes, *more* filthy lucre. Don't neglect other media—audiobooks, videos, CDs—which can easily be resold or donated.

If you're looking for something to read, libraries are a bargain for you and the planet. Used-book stores are a close second. If you don't live near a well-stocked secondhand bookshop, you can search for used books through your favorite online book retailer or check out Bookfinder (www.bookfinder.com).

Last, when you're finished with *this* book, consider passing it on to a friend. Really. We would gladly give up our royalties for the sake of the planet. And if you happen to know a good accountant, kindly let me know. Ours just quit.

CHAPTER 5

MONEY, CREDIT, AND INVESTING

It is truly enough said that a corporation has no conscience; but a corporation of conscientious men is a corporation with a conscience.
—HENRY DAVID THOREAU

Ironically, money can compete with living a good life. While very useful for the exchange of goods and services, it may be the single biggest cause of our alienation from nature. To be more specific, money itself may not be to blame, but our relationship to it certainly dominates how our institutions operate. Well, I have some news: the almighty and somewhat dysfunctional dollar provides great opportunity for change and influence. In America we are consumers—and therein lies a great deal of power.

I'd like to see a completely new true-cost accounting system that would represent natural resources—including the well-being of the citizens of this planet. The health of our population, our air, our water, and the species sharing this planet are not currently represented on America's bottom line. Instead we look to our gross national product (GNP), which indicates how much money is moving through our economy, to judge whether things are going well. This is a good measure of the wealth and quantity of "stuff" being produced and consumed in our economy—but it doesn't account for well-being and health. We are focusing on the results, not the process, and there is no indication that the results will arrive looking any better than last night's pizza.

The Iroquois Nations made all decisions with respect to the impact in seven generations' time. Think about the introduction of DDT in 1942. Under a fifty-year plan the question as to where the forty million tons of insecticide would ultimately reside after application would have been raised and addressed. Might the peregrine falcon have been spared the risk of extinction? And humans spared the risk of exposure to toxins?

Whether you own a home, have stocks and savings, or live in a VW bus with a view of a surf break, you do not have to wholly participate in a consumer culture. You can pick investments that are environmentally and ecologically sound. You can buy products from corporations that respect your values. You can incorporate the basic principles of voluntary simplicity, carefully scrutinizing your needs and only choosing to buy things that add real value to your life. You might buy satellite Internet service and forgo owning a car. The key is deciding what is appropriate and necessary for you. My friend and teacher Joseph Goldstein once said, "Think of all the pleasurable experiences you've ever had in your lifetime. Where are they now?" I don't mean to imply that pleasure isn't worth seeking, but remember that pleasure isn't permanent. We can step off the proverbial treadmill, acknowledge consumer gratifications are fleeting, and begin working toward joy, a condition that accepts the true nature of change, and for which there is no upgraded version.

I realize I'm in the thick of it when I look at the stuff I have: my computer, my car, and my favorite surfboards. I am not prepared, honestly, to give these things up. I do believe, however, that business is one of the most influential means of change, and how we influence business—through our consumerism—is one of our best opportunities to encourage conscientious action.

Sixty-one percent of Americans invest in the stock market. Fifty million households own mutual funds, to the tune of $27 trillion. Americans have a powerful tool for righting wrong, and it's as close to us as our wallets and checkbooks.

Much of the money in the stock market is invested conventionally. In other words, investors chase profit and profit alone. But a different kind of investor is emerging. It doesn't matter what you call this investor—socially conscious, socially responsible, ethical, natural, or faith-based—whatever the sobriquet, the strategy is the same. This investor still hankers for profit but chooses investments according to personal values. Screening stocks this way *can* affect the market. Companies deemed profitable—and good corporate citizens—will thrive on Wall Street. Bad corporate citizens won't.

Not all mutual-fund companies have the energy or desire to get involved in conscientious investing, but a small segment of the fund universe regards it as their mission. There are activists even on Wall Street. In fact, 2001 was one of the busiest years for picking fights with major corporations. With the blessing of their investors, the people who manage these portfolios fought to abolish sweatshops, railed against genetically modified organisms that threaten our food supply, and pushed companies to promote more women and minorities to leadership positions.

Suddenly we've all got another good reason to invest.

But every day, in little ways, each of us supports and subsidizes large corporations. A swipe of your credit card enriches not only the store you're buying from but also a credit-card provider, a bank, or both. When you whip out the ATM card, you send a clear signal that you have chosen one financial institution over another. At every stage, someone is taking a small cut. Don't you wish you could hand those fees over to people who will do some good with them?

These days you can. A growing number of credit cards share profits with charities and environmental groups. And certain types of financial institutions are devoted to investing in local economies.

I hope the next few pages will challenge you to start thinking about who profits from your credit card, banking, and investment money. And I'd like to inspire you to use your money to benefit three important entities—yourself, your immediate community, and the world you live in.

THE NEW BENCHMARK

Sometimes a revolution begins with a suggestion, a complaint, a lament. That's how it was for Amy Domini. In the early eighties she worked as a stockbroker and was privileged to witness how her clients' convictions sometimes bubbled up to the surface and shaped their finances. Some clients asked her to keep their portfolios free of tobacco-company stocks. An avid birdwatcher was targeting a paper company that was clear-cutting forests. Another instructed her to steer clear of military contractors.

Amy was sympathetic to these requests. She was a product of her culture and times. As the daughter of an immigrant father, she had grown up longing for social justice and equality. When she was in her teens, her grandfather taught her how to read annual reports, all the while railing against the outrageous salaries company bosses paid themselves. She grew up witnessing the fight for civil rights and protests against the Vietnam War. She took all these lessons to heart, and eventually found herself working on Wall Street.

> *Somebody's gotta keep an eye on these big geniuses.*
> *—Judy Holliday, in* **The Solid Gold Cadillac** *(1956)*

She knew that, historically, people had often tied their livelihoods to their beliefs. In the 1690s Quaker settlers in Pennsylvania denounced slavery and vowed not to encourage or profit from the sale of other human beings. In the 1980s investors who divested their portfolios of any business profiting from the apartheid system instigated major change in South Africa.

Despite the precedent, plenty of Wall Streeters thought then—and still think—that the goals of social investing are wrong-headed. "They say investing is the wrong place to bring ethics," Amy, now fifty-two, says today. "But like it or not, investing has built the world we live in. And somebody's ethics are already embedded in the practices of major corporations. So in other words, those ethics are accelerating global warming. Or personal injuries might result from those ethics. These is no nonethical investing."

Amy knew that if social investing was going to take off, it had to demolish its biggest hurdle: the notion that you couldn't make money doing it. In the late eighties she and two colleagues, Peter Kinder and Steve Lydenberg, began constructing a financial index called the Domini 400 Social Index. It was modeled after well-known indices such as Standard & Poor's 500. To make an index, you simply pick a collection of stocks and monitor their prices minute by minute, hour by hour, day by day. And this helps you gauge how well the market is doing.

Amy, Peter, and Steve created the Domini 400 out of companies that fall into one of two categories. For the first, they drew up lists of companies that didn't profit from the sale of alcohol, tobacco, gambling, nuclear power, or military contracts. Then they combed through each of them, keeping companies that had a good environmental impact as well as good citizenship, employee relations, and diversity. As it turned out, about half of the Standard & Poor's 500 companies qualified for the Domini 400 in the trio's first go-round. Then they added 150 new companies that reflected the market's diversity and were particularly strong models of corporate behavior. Today the Domini 400's top ten holdings include Coca-Cola, Cisco Systems, SBC Communications, Verizon, Merck, Johnson & Johnson, Intel, American International Group, AOL Time Warner, and Microsoft. Some of these companies still have a long way to go, but thoughtful investing allows you to positively influence large companies whose policies fall short of the ideal. Corporations recognize both their customers and their investors and will go to great lengths to please both. As an investor, you can lobby for change within the system.

As they were designing the index, Amy and her colleagues wondered just how profitable this collection of companies would be in the months and years ahead. Would it hold its own against the S&P? They thought it would. It seemed to make sense that if a company worked hard at being a good corporate citizen, it would probably avoid lawsuits and scandal. It turns out they were right. The ten-year track record shows that picking stocks this way is no worse than putting your faith in the S&P 500. In fact, the Domini 400 Social Index has outperformed the S&P 500 on a cumulative basis.

The industry Amy helped create is growing each year. Besides her own mutual-fund company, Domini Social Investments, there are about 180 funds in the United States that screen stocks using varying degrees and kinds of criteria. And similar funds are now available in countries around the world. Of these, the best are those that work actively to file shareholder resolutions and support community banks. Now, you can certainly skip mutual funds and buy stocks on your own if you are a highly motivated investor. But it's easier to bring pressure upon a wayward company if you do it in numbers. Activist mutual funds, with their huge numbers and dollars, can more effectively infiltrate the corporations and force a dialogue. If they accomplish these two things, says Amy, they'll accomplish something deeper.

> *What is the strongest force on the planet? It's you and your investment account and me with my investment account. What I'm arguing about here is that, at some fundamental level, the people that move the money move society. We need to take responsibility for that impact. The way you make money makes a difference.*
> —*Amy Domini*

"I believe a healthy society is one that is created by healthy people," she says. "A social investor subtly alters his or her sense of self. You don't feel helpless. You're glad the fund is doing something about the problems. You feel part of the solution.

"I'll tell you a little story. I started going to an organic market when it opened in Cambridge, Massachusetts, where I live. I went a couple of times and bought the food and read the signs in the aisles about the importance of eating organic. As you read the signs, you start to become political. By the third time I went there I started to think of myself as a freedom fighter. I knew I was making a difference. What I'm saying is that the first step in any recovery is hope. Social investing gives people hope. It's a way to address real problems in the world today. It works because a mutual fund is not one person putting millions of dollars into a fund. It's millions of people putting a dollar into it. And they all feel more empowered."

MONEY,
CREDIT,
AND INVESTING

CASH AND CONSCIENCE

A woman I'll call Staci was only a few years out of school when she began to empower herself this way. She'd grown up in a progressive family. Her parents were Depression-era leftists, and Staci took their sensibilities to heart. In college she was politically active, and when she left school she saw no reason to abandon her idealism.

When one of her relatives passed away, Staci was stunned to learn she had inherited some serious cash.

"It was a strange convergence," she says today, almost twenty years later. "Political activism and money seemed to me like two things that didn't mesh well."

The money made her feel uncomfortable. Her parents had always been fiscally conservative. As children of tougher times, they thought the only place for money was a safe place. Only the rich dabbled in the stock market, and look what a mess they'd made of the world while doing it.

> *Money is of no value; it cannot spend itself. All depends on the skill of the spender.*
> —*Ralph Waldo Emerson*

After mulling it over, Staci decided to follow in her parents' footsteps. She'd make a conservative investment. She remembers going to a bank and filling out the forms to buy U.S. Treasury notes. She handed her paperwork over the counter to the teller, who stopped and said, "With this kind of money, you should be buying real estate. You'd make more money than buying treasuries."

Staci hesitated. It was clear she'd have to put more thought into this whole money thing. This was in the days when socially responsible investing was a fairly hidden phenomenon, and there weren't many books on the topic. Staci did her homework. Treasuries funded the U.S. government, which funded the military, but mortgage-backed bonds such as Fannie Maes didn't. Pretty soon these bonds formed the backbone of her portfolio.

She chuckles about it today. "Considering what I knew at the time," she says, "I don't think I did badly."

Eventually, Staci sought out the services of a like-minded broker. It helped to find someone who was on the same wavelength:

a guy who enjoyed the challenge of finding stocks and bonds that were appropriate fits for his clients. These days Staci does very little researching work. "I just give him the screens," she says. "I tell him I don't want to invest in the military or military contractors. No oil. No union-busting companies. No animal research. And yes to any companies with progressive policies for women."

You'd think with those kinds of limits her investments would not have budged. But that's not the case. One of her friends—a stock advisor who thinks socially responsible investing (SRI) means backing shaky soy-milk companies—always used to mock her. But that all ended the day he innocently inquired what her rate of return was and got the shock of his life.

At forty-three, Staci doesn't think she's lost anything investing this way. She wouldn't dream of giving up what feels like a natural way to invest her money.

Her only caveat to newcomers: be open to change. Socially invested stocks are just as volatile as those you invest in using financial criteria alone. "I invested early on in a company that got through all my screens and has done very well. But just the other day I saw in the newspaper that they're in trouble for labor-relations problems. It just shows you. Things develop."

DEFINING THE TERMS

True social investing is accomplished by using three different strategies:

Screening. All investing requires a screen—a criterion or set of criteria that helps you determine which companies' stocks will be included in a portfolio and which will be excluded. Socially responsible investors choose stocks, bonds, mutual funds, and other instruments according to social or environmental screens. They may, for example, choose not to invest in companies that profit from alcohol, tobacco, gambling, nuclear power, or petroleum products. Others may screen out companies known to test their products on animals, pollute the environment, or manufacture weapons.

Shareholder activism. When you buy stock, you become part owner in a company. Socially responsible investors use their clout—enormous clout in the case of mutual funds that own millions of shares of a particular company—to propose shareholder resolutions and force companies to negotiate or vote on important issues.

Community investment. These days multinational corporations know no boundaries. The world is their oyster (and no one else's). Therein lies their strength—and their greatest failing. Socially responsible investors reward banks, credit unions, and small businesses that work hard to improve life in local economies. They may also invest in municipal bonds that fund public initiatives.

- Almost one out of every eight dollars under management in the United States today is part of a socially responsible portfolio.

- Tobacco-company stocks are the ones investors most often choose to avoid.

- More than $900 billion in assets are used to lobby corporations through shareholder advocacy.

(Source: *2001 Trends Report,* Social Investment Forum)

WHAT YOU CAN DO

Here are some ways you can make a difference in the way you manage your money.

Get your priorities straight. Before you subscribe to mountains of personal-finance magazines or become addicted to advice talk shows, get your finances in order. Every credible money guru offers this excellent advice: don't invest a dime speculatively until you get yourself out of debt and have an emergency fund stashed away. How much? Three to six months' living expenses, at minimum, stockpiled in a low-risk investment such as a bank money-market account or bank certificates of deposit.

Any exceptions? Well, okay, there are a few. During this time, when you are paying down your debt, you may invest in retirement savings accounts (such as Roth IRAs, 401(k) plans, Keogh, and profit-sharing plans) which, except for special circumstances, you won't be able to touch until you retire. If you have children, don't neglect Coverdell education savings accounts (CESAs), UGMA/UTMAs, and state-sponsored 529 plans. All of these instruments allow your money to grow tax-free, so you'd be wise to avail yourself of them. And by all means, consider making these social investments. In all but one of these accounts, that won't be a problem. As we go to press, only two states—California and Pennsylvania—are offering a social-investment opportunity as part of their 529 plan.

> *Without prosperous local economies, the people have no power, and the land no voice.*
> —*Wendell Berry*

Use a socially responsible credit card. I know, I know. What's so responsible about more consumption, more packaging, more trash, more stuff you probably don't need? Indeed, you can help the planet more by saving your money and making regular donations to the charities or environmental groups of your choice. But if you are going to spend the money anyway—on grocery shopping, gas, dentist bills—choose a credit card that donates a portion of its profits to a worthwhile cause, or is issued by a credit union or small bank known for its community investment. Before you sign up, scrutinize the fine print. Some companies donate nothing, but the design of their card—soaring eagles, furry bear cubs—leads you believe they do. The best known, Working Assets (www.workingassets.com/creditcard), donates ten cents of every purchase to one of numerous causes. Cards are also available through Alternatives Federal Credit Union (www.alternatives.org/visacard.html), First Savings of New Hampshire "Card for Kids" (www.chittenden.com/newfsnh/per-srb.html), First USA (www.firstusa.com), and the Giving Card (www.thegivingcard.com).

Use a community-development bank or credit union. Most of us pick our banks the way we pick supermarkets. The one closest to home wins, or the one with the most ATMs. Smaller financial

Dispelling the Myths

MYTH: Socially responsible investing is just not profitable.

FACT: KLD, the Boston research firm that created the Domini 400, says it has found no correlation between a portfolio's ethics and its performance over the long term. In its first ten years, the Domini 400 Social Index has returned an average of 13.77 percent compared with 12.95 percent for the S&P 500. The stock market is inherently volatile, but a diversified portfolio should be able to ride out the ups and downs. It's the long haul that counts, cowboy.

MYTH: Socially responsible companies have higher expenses. So do the mutual funds that invest in them.

FACT: Who's calling the kettle black? Yes, it may cost more to institute fair labor practices or conscientious environmental programs. But these eliminate surprises for shareholders later on down the road. Fewer nasty lawsuits, fewer product recalls, no embarrassing environmental disasters, no bad publicity, and no stomach-churning drops in stock value. Socially screened mutual funds may have high expense ratios due to the amount of research that must go into them. But managers says those costs will likely drop as corporations become more accountable, and more transparent, to their shareholders.

MYTH: Using social values to screen investments limits choice.

FACT: So what? All investing is an exercise in limited choice. You can't invest in everything. Mutual-fund managers, for example, select stocks, bonds, and other instruments according to criteria consistent with a specific fund's goals. Large-cap funds invest in big companies, small-caps in small ones, and municipal-bond funds eschew corporate and treasury bonds. For that matter, most folks on Wall Street are experts in a single investment category or market sector. They're not so much masters of the universe as they are petty viceroys of the planet Cashola.

> **MYTH:** It's impossible to have a company that's 100 percent "clean."
>
> **FACT:** Okay, this time we agree. It's worth repeating again and again so your delusions of perfection are suitably dashed. No matter how squeaky clean a company is, it's impossible to eliminate all threats to humanity and the environment in the work you do. (I ought to know.) Simply by existing, a company consumes the earth's precious resources. The point is, you've got to keep trying because the effort you expend, in part, defines the company (or person) you are.

institutions, such as credit unions and community banks, have a better track record of investing in local communities and providing loans to people and businesses other banks consider unbankable. "If a bank has only two branches," says Amy Domini, "chances are good that the money they lend out is going back into your hometown." If you're shopping for a loan, a new bank, or a place to park some money in a CD, you might consider one of these institutions. Traditional credit unions are members-only, but many, like the Self-Help Credit Union (www.self-help.org), let you join for a small (in this case, twenty-five dollars) annual fee. To find other credit unions, see the Resources Directory.

Get to know yourself first. You want to take this socially responsible business in easy steps. It makes sense to spend some time figuring out where your values lie. Are you primarily interested in supporting companies that work toward a sustainable environment and avoiding ones that don't? Are you also interested in social issues such as labor relations, workplace discrimination, and sweatshop reform? Are alcohol, tobacco, gambling, and weapons on your hit list? Do you have religious beliefs that shape the way you invest? These types of questions can help identify the screens important to you.

Get to know the stocks you already own. If you already have a sizable portfolio and you're concerned that you may have invested in lots of questionable companies, you'll go nuts (and possibly

Selecting Screens

Socially responsible investors may regard these issues as undesirable in an investment:

Alcohol

Animal testing

Child labor

Environmental pollution

Gambling

Global warming

High executive pay

Military contractors

Nuclear power

Oppressive governments abroad

Poor hiring of women and minorities

Sweatshops

Tobacco

Workplace discrimination

Socially responsible investors may regard these issues as desirable in an investment:

Community development

Conservation

Diversity in board of directors
   and employees

Education

Encouraging or building
   affordable housing

Environmental cleanup

Fair wages, human rights, and
   environmental concern in
   businesses abroad

Progressive workplace policies

Recycling

Safe products and services

Using or making tree substitutes

Using or creating clean transportation
   technologies

Using or providing renewable energy

broke) if you start buying and selling recklessly. The best way to proceed is to visit Social Funds (www.socialfunds.com) and Social Investment Forum (www.socialinvest.org), the two best websites devoted to SRI. If you already have assets, draw up a list of what you own and spend some time learning how each company holds up to socially responsible screening. Folks who do this for a living have access to expensive research reports on various companies, but there are other ways to find out how a company stacks up.

- Read the company's annual report (it's usually puffery, but you can still learn a lot) and a recent proxy statement (the one printed on flimsy white paper). This will tell you how much money the bigwigs are earning as well as provide info on the retirement plans and any action a company is contemplating at its next meeting. You'll also learn whether some socially responsible investors are calling for a vote on an important topic.

- If you own mutual funds, you can find out the fund manager's rationale for selecting a specific stock at that fund's website. To make it easy on yourself, you might want to scrutinize only the top ten holdings in each fund. You can also study the top holdings of some of the funds we list in our funds chart.

- A quick search at Domini Funds (www.domini.com) or KLD (www.kld.com) will tell you if a company is part of the Domini 400 or if Domini or KLD has recently blown the whistle on a company's questionable practices. Calvert (www.calvert.com/sri_calvertindex.asp) has a similar searchable index. CorpWatch (www.corpwatch.org), a watchdog site, summarizes outstanding shareholder actions against corporations. SRI News (www.srinews.com) keeps tabs on what's happening in the industry. *Green Money Journal* (www.greenmoney.com) monitors SRI developments.

- You can read up on companies the usual way—through the news media.

Vote the stocks you have. A lot of us ignore proxies when they come in the mail. But these little slips of paper represent the best way to change a corporation from the inside. In recent years, the managers of socially invested mutual funds have sought amendments to corporate policies on a host of issues. When these resolutions come to a vote, they usually fail to pass. But a company will do almost anything to avoid an embarrassing proxy fight. It's this delicious arm-twisting that brings plenty of corporations to the negotiation table. So from now on, if you receive a proxy mentioning a "shareholder resolution," read up on the issue and then vote your conscience. You can also write a letter to companies you're targeting at Social Funds (www.socialfunds.com) or Shareholder Action (www.shareholderaction.org).

Choose a broker or financial planner who understands. If your assets are considerable or just complicated, you may benefit from using a broker or financial planner. Finding one who's fluent in the socially responsible movement is not as difficult as it used to be, since the market for this type of investing has grown. Social Funds (www.social funds.com) and Good Money (www.goodmoney .com/directry_pros.htm) offer searchable lists of prospects, so you can easily locate someone in your neck of the woods. It's nice to find a person who shares your politics, but remember that these folks are not necessarily your chums. Full-service brokers earn a hefty commission for every transaction they make on your behalf. On top of that, brokerage accounts carry annual maintenance fees. A financial planner either charges a flat rate for advice or takes a commission on transactions.

Or do it yourself. If you've done your homework, there's no reason why you can't handle your own investments. It's certainly cheaper. By one estimate, discount brokerages charge one twentieth what full-service brokers do. Some of the bigger discount houses include Ameritrade (www.ameritrade.com), Datek (www.datek .com), Brown & Co. (www.brownco3.com), Harris Direct (www.harrisdirect.com), and TD Waterhouse (www.tdwater house.com). Instead of buying stock in pricey lots of fifty or one hundred shares—one of the biggest hurdles for small investors—

you can also buy shares of mutual funds, or individual stock in fractional amounts. Both FOLIO*fn* (www.foliofn.com) and Sharebuilder (www.sharebuilder.com) specialize in this type of investing. FOLIO*fn* lets customers invest in preselected portfolios, including five shaped with social issues in mind.

SAMPLE PORTFOLIO

Many people have the idea that social investing means putting your trust and your money in small, unknown companies. Nothing could be further from the truth. Here's a glimpse at one of FOLIO*fn*'s "ready-to-go" portfolios. This environmentally responsible portfolio is described as "a Folio of companies that have no toxic emissions, oil and chemical spills, or compliance penalties, and have not recently been identified as potentially responsible for Superfund sites."

American International
  Group Inc.
Allstate Corp.
Amgen Inc.
American Express Co.
Bank of America Corp.
Bank New York Inc.
Cisco Systems Inc.
Dell Computer Corp.
Fleetboston Financial Corp.
First Data Corp.
Fifth Third Bancorp.
Federal National Mortgage
  Assn.
Federal Home Loan
  Mortgage Corp.
Home Depot Inc.
J. P. Morgan Chase & Co.

MBNA Corp.
Kohls Corp.
Lowes Cos. Inc.
Marsh & McLennan Cos. Inc.
Microsoft Corp.
Morgan Stanley Dean Witter
  & Co.
Bank One Corp.
Oracle Corp.
Tenet Healthcare Corp.
United Health Group
US Bancorp Del.
Wachovia Corp.
Wells Fargo & Co.
Washington Mutual
Wal-Mart Stores

Socially Responsible Mutual Funds

Here's a sampling of some of the respected social funds on the market. All the ones on this list screen stocks. Commitment to shareholder activism and community investing varies from fund to fund.

CALVERT (www.calvertgroup.com)

Capital Accumulation	Social Equity
Large Cap Growth	Social Index
New Vision Small Cap	Social Technology
Social Balanced	World Values International
Social Bond	Equity
Social Enhanced Equity	Social Money Market

DOMINI (www.domini.com)

Social Bond	Money Market
Social Equity	

GREEN CENTURY (www.greencentury.com)

Balanced	Equity

MMA PRAXIS (www.mmapraxis.com)

Core Stock	International
Intermediate Income	Value Index

NEW ALTERNATIVES (www.newalternativesfund.com)

PARNASSUS (www.parnassus.com)

California Tax-Free	Fixed Income
Equity Income	Fund

PAX WORLD (www.paxfund.com)

Fund	High-Yield Bond
Growth	Money Market

PORTFOLIO 21 (www.portfolio21.com)

WALDEN (www.waldenassetmgmt.com)

Social Balanced	B&BT Domestic Social Index
Social Equity	B&BT International Social Index

ONE LAST WORD . . .

When you look at how much money is being invested in this country, you'd think we were all a savvy bunch of investors, people who really knew the value of a nickel, dime, or dollar. But that's not really so. As much as we want what money can do for us, we don't really understand it.

But each dollar you earn and send into the world is your ambassador, because time has been shaved off your life to get it. If you start thinking of money this way, you'll want to invest as wisely as possible. You'll try to make your investments say as much about you as the car you drive or the foods you eat. And on that note, no, we don't sell stock in our company, but it never hurts to invest in a few pretzels.

CHAPTER 6

SHOPPING

They came, they saw, they did a little shopping.
—GRAFFITI ON THE BERLIN WALL,
AFTER THE FALL

I recently pulled off the highway en route from San Francisco to Santa Cruz, into the parking lot of what I'll call my local Mega-Mart. I parked behind a VW bus circa 1968 adorned with no fewer than thirty-three bumper stickers. The two most prominent read: FRANK ZAPPA FOR PRESIDENT and THINK GLOBALLY, ACT LOCALLY. If this bus isn't broken down, it has no business being in the parking lot of a national chain store. On second thought, what business do I have here? What am I shopping for that I cannot do without? Whatever it was, the bumper stickers have me completely distracted.

There is something unsettling in the concept of thinking globally and acting locally. Mega-Mart is thinking globally. The petroleum industry is thinking globally. Am I acting locally by walking into Mega-Mart, or am I supporting global enterprise?

America, open for business. Shopping, we are being told, is now a form of patriotism. During World War II our nation was asked to conserve, save, and plant a victory garden. Today I feel like I'm being asked to play in a shopping tournament. For America to win, I need to support all these global corporations who will in turn support limitless economic growth. Economic growth, which depends on unimpeded trade channels, is thought to demonstrate that the American way is good and right. A plunger! That's what I needed.

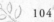

It is astonishing how much merchandise a Mega-Mart contains—halogen lights, cutting boards, big plastic storage boxes. Have you ever wondered how this stuff can be so inexpensive? How a halogen lamp manufactured in China, packed in Styrofoam, cardboard, and cellophane, and shipped to California can sell for $14.99? What is the hidden cost associated with all these cheap goods? And what evidence really demonstrates that the answer to our global problems is more free-market economies? Is consumerism a reasonable and sane means to health for our local economies, our neighborhoods, and our personal well-being?

Well, I have a theory about consumer gratification. It has something to do with wealth being more than money, and value being more than the price of something. It has to do with whatever might cause a shopper to pause and question what appears to be a great bargain but on closer inspection entails, in a far part of the globe, abuse of a resource. It has to do with a concept called "fair trade" that promotes and ensures responsible use of resources and fair treatment of workers. In my experience, and perhaps in yours too, buying fair-trade products leads to real customer satisfaction.

How about these bumper stickers? CONSPICUOUS CONSUMPTION JUST MAKES YOU MORE CONSPICUOUS. THINK BEFORE YOU BUY, YOU MIGHT BE REINCARNATED AS A THIRD-WORLD LABORER. IF HAPPINESS IS FLEETING, WHY ARE YOU PAYING FOR IT IN FOUR EASY INSTALLMENTS? GUMPTION BEFORE CONSUMPTION.

Did I buy the plunger or not? Well, at the end of this musing, I still needed one. But I was reminded that shopping is an influential and powerful means of expression. My actions at the cash register are significant. And so it is with these and other great bumper stickers in mind that I share with you a few ideas about being a cash-register activist. And I'm sure if Frank Zappa were alive and were president, his reactions to a politically and economically fragile climate wouldn't be a call for everyone to go shopping. He might, perhaps, write a song about a giant rubber plunger that could unclog bad foreign-policy buildup.

CASH-REGISTER CLOUT

To live is to consume. But we can make a change for the better by thinking twice about our purchases. Shoppers wield enormous clout. You, with your dollars waiting to be spent, have the ear of corporations and manufacturers. In order to make their goods and services attractive to you, they will do almost anything to please. Notice how much money they spend trying to woo you and keep you.

When you choose to buy natural, nontoxic products, you are stating that your family's health—and the health of the soil and waterways—matters to you. When you shift your dollars from a megastore to a mom-and-pop because the smaller place carries water-soluble paint and decking that isn't loaded with arsenic, you're showing the big boys the way to your heart and you're supporting your local economy too. If a company hasn't been a good neighbor—they recklessly pollute the city where they're headquartered, they refuse to recycle, or they won't give their workers a fair shake—you can withhold your dollars from them until they shape up.

> ## It All Adds Up
>
> 25 percent disposable income of $40,000 per year, over 40 years = $400,000

This kind of activism has a wonderful ripple effect. Because each time you spend a buck, you're likely to spend wisely, waste less, and educate others by your example. I recall that one Christmas my father stuffed our stockings with bizarre wooden trinkets—a couple of tiny dowels inserted into a flat base—and then sat back to watch me, my sisters, and our mom try to figure out what they were. Finally, with perverse glee, he gave it up: they were plastic-bag dryers! Each time you used a plastic bag, instead of tossing it, you could rinse it, dry it, and use it again. We made much fun of his dorky present . . . but we use them still.

That's just a small example, but it speaks volumes. It's great to recycle, but it's even better to *reduce* and *reuse* our waste. Much of the stuff we buy defies modern recycling efforts. If it's not an easily classified material such as paper, glass, or aluminum, it gets a one-way ticket to the dump. The ancient Egyptians built pyramids that endure to this day. Our culture is building landfills. For centuries the Great Wall of China was the largest manmade structure on earth. Astronauts could spot it from the moon. About a decade ago the Great Wall became dwarfed by the Fresh Kills Landfill—a now-closed dump that served New York City since the 1940s. This "peak" is the highest geographic feature along a fifteen-hundred-mile stretch of the Atlantic seaboard running north from Florida all the way to Maine.

We used to think that everything in a landfill simply rotted away. Now we know that's not true. If anything, the objects are preserved. Mummified, if you will. Scientists have excavated thirty-year-old phone books—that are perfectly legible—from dumps. Though the people who run these sites take pains to contain the effluent that oozes from them, the chance that the runoff may pollute groundwater is always a concern.

So don't ever let anyone tell you your shopping habits don't matter. Purchases are intentional acts that can either harm or help. To get you started, I've highlighted some of the major concerns in the sections that follow and suggested some earth-friendly sources. (Check out the Resources Directory at the back of the book for addresses and other information.)

Clothing

Cotton is grown on 3 to 5 percent of the world's cultivated lands—but is sprayed with 25 percent of the world's pesticide each year. If that isn't bad enough, the fashion industry is notorious for sending its contracts overseas and turning a blind eye to sweatshop practices.

At this time, there are no federal guidelines governing organic clothing. Only the fibers themselves—the agricultural products, in other words—can be certified organic. Conscientious makers like Maggie's will insist on harmless dyes, threads, and other supplies that end up in finished products. Since workplace practices

Sewing What They Reap

Bená Burda has been selling organic-cotton clothing since the early nineties. Her signature items are comfy organic-cotton socks, but she also sells T-shirts, camisoles, and other great stuff through her company, Maggie's Organics. "I got into this to save acreage," she says. "At the time, even people in the organic-food industry didn't know how bad the cotton situation was." In 1998 Bená Burda was searching desperately for a factory to stitch some of her organic-cotton products. She was determined not to patronize a sweatshop that exploited workers. She heard about Jubilee House—a refugee center in Nicaragua with many willing and able workers—and asked, "Can they sew?"

When a group of about twenty women said they could or would be willing to learn, Burda worked the phones from Ann Arbor, locating a batch of used sewing machines the women could buy on the cheap. Jubilee House arranged for a parcel of land, building materials, and some cash to buy the equipment. These efforts were a great start, but they were nothing compared with what the refugee women did next.

Over the next two years, they literally built the factory themselves. At the same time, they established a sophisticated vestment program; in essence, those who helped build would reap a share of the profits later on. They also pledged to set aside funds to help develop other local businesses.

Burda has been delighted by the quality of their work, and she has the satisfaction of knowing that her products are environmentally sustainable and promote quality of life in a developing nation.

are difficult to assess, you should patronize companies that disclose how they gauge a factory's practices. Part of the Maggie's line is created by a women's sewing cooperative in Nicaragua; those who sew share in all profits. So the dollars you spend on a Maggie's T-shirt help both land and people. Not bad.

If you are concerned about the use of leather—because of either the animal issue or the strong chemicals used in tanning—consider switching to footwear using hemp fabrics and recycled rubber. Manmade leather is another option but may generate a similarly harmful waste stream. Don't discount vintage clothing; it's stylish and has already paid its debt to the planet.

Toys

The biggest issue in toys is the use of chemicals called phthalates, which soften plastic. Phthalates can leach from products, especially when kids or pets suck, nibble, or chew on them. The issue is still controversial, debated hotly by activists, legislators, and manufacturers. If you are concerned, choose PVC-free toys and pacifiers. Beyond this issue, environmentally conscious parents try to reduce their child's exposure to toxins in baby products, bedding, childhood furniture, paints, and window treatments. Parents of older kids may look for games, toys, and reading materials that encourage cooperative gaming, respect for human dignity, and environmental sustainability.

Gifts

Selecting fine gifts for people you respect or love is one of life's great pleasures. Low-impact gifts like certificates to movies, restaurants, and spas generate no waste. I encourage you to shop locally for special organic goods—wines, cheeses, honeys—and patronize artisans of sustainable crafts. Some organizations, such as SERRV, sell handmade products that benefit craftspeople in developing nations. The fair-trade movement, which guarantees workers in developing nations a living wage, is an excellent way to give gifts that support these goals.

Home Building Supplies and Furnishings

When I first moved out West, I found a newly built house to rent. As the move-in date approached, I went out to visit the place and got a shock. The builders had just finished painting and the air reeked of noxious odors. Inside, the wall-to-wall carpeting, appliances, and newly varnished floors were all giving off a myriad of fumes. Out in the backyard, they'd left a small patch of dirt to use as a garden. Unfortunately, it was filled with time-release herbicides used to kill weeds as they sprout. Although I knew all of this had been done with the best of intentions, I just couldn't see myself living there. I eventually found a place that suited my needs.

Potentially harmful toxins lurk in products such as fiberglass, adhesives, paints, finishes, strippers—and that's just the beginning. The powerful odors left behind by paint jobs and installations represent what is known in the industry as volatile organic compounds (VOCs). Here's a simple rule of thumb: if you smell them, they're getting into your lungs. Besides the structure of your home, seemingly benign furnishings such as sofas and mattresses have been known to irritate skin. Pressure-treated lumber, the ubiquitous deck-building material, is impregnated with arsenic to resist rot and water damage. Luckily, a number of contractors and companies sell products, like those made from sustainably harvested lumber, that won't harm you or the environment. Your purchase helps the communities where these products are made stay healthy.

Cosmetics and Baby Products

Aubrey Hampton, a pioneer in organic beauty products, grew up on an Indiana farm, learning how to make natural creams, shampoos, and lotions from his mother, a self-taught herbalist. "My brother used to help her out too," Aubrey recalls. "But he spilled things. So he ended up working on the farm with my dad, and I helped my mom." Aubrey, who longed to be a playwright, worked in New York City theater in the early fifties, about the same time my parents were getting their start. Since money was tight, he made his own soaps and shampoos out of natural ingredients such as chamomile, lavender, and aloe. Pretty soon he was selling his wares in health-food stores.

He was ahead of his time. Then, as now, manufacturers are allowed to use petroleum-based synthetic fragrances, dyes, and chemicals to create their products. No one seemed to worry about what these concoctions would do to a customer's skin or hair after years of use. If it didn't cause someone immediate harm, it was okay. To ensure short-term safety, companies tested everything on animals. This outraged Aubrey. "I grew up on a farm," he says. "I knew how animals should be treated. They all have a life. On a farm you take care of animals because you know, ultimately, they take care of you."

The cosmetics industry continues to be woefully underregulated. You should read the labels of all personal-care products— soaps, shampoos, toothpastes, lip balms, beauty products, sunblock, sexual lubricants, literally anything that touches or enters your body—regardless of their source. Products that are billed as "natural" or "hypoallergenic" may be as likely as conventional products to have negative long-term effects. In recent years environmental groups have advocated limiting exposure to a number of chemicals in personal-care products—such as DEA, TEA, bronopol, padimate-O, ethoxylated alcohols, 1,4-dioxane, artificial colors and fragrances, and formaldehyde—believed to cause dermatitis or cancer. The universe of consumer products is vast and changing, but if you take the time to read labels and do a little research from time to time, you'll develop a more mindful shopping routine, one that allows you to feel good about what you buy.

What You Can Do

Observe the cardinal rule. Buy not what you want but what you need. Anytime you buy anything, more of the earth's resources are consumed. There's more trash to toss out. More fossil fuels consumed to make the object, wrap it, and get it to your home. More pollution is created. It helps to cultivate the habit of thinking before you spend. You might want to ask yourself questions such as:

Do I really need it?
Can I reuse something to get the same job done?
Can I repair something I now own?
Can I buy a used, vintage, or recycled version?
Are there any manufacturers I should avoid?
Are there any socially or environmentally responsible manufacturers
    I can support?

Spend time and energy before dollars and fuel. The Internet is the perfect tool for researching stores, prices, and product features. If you have your heart set on a juicer with vacuum attachments, a Web search will reveal that standard parts will be in short

Who Cares About Green Consuming?

- Fifty-three percent of Americans say they have bought a product because the advertising or label said it was environmentally safe or biodegradable.

- Fifty percent say they're willing to pay more for earth-friendly products.

- Fifty percent say they would do more for the environment but don't know how.

(Source: Roper Green Gauge Report)

supply for as long as you own it. Your local library will also have back issues of *Consumer Reports,* longtime friend of anyone itching to spend.

Be choosy about how you vote with your dollars. Before you spend your money on a product, you might want to research its safety or its manufacturer's social or environmental record. Responsible Shopper (www.responsibleshopper.org) will help with the latter. *The Safe Shopper's Bible,* by David Steinman and

Samuel S. Epstein, M.D. (Macmillan, 1995), ranks thousands of home products according to attributes such as skin sensitivity and carcinogenity. As you read up, you'll begin to identify your own values. Following are some positive qualities you might want in a product or choose to support through your shopping. Don't let the list intimidate you. These attributes are intended only as a guide.

- All-natural: Contains no hormones, artificial flavorings, colorings, or preservatives.

- Chemical sensitivity safe: Contains no synthetic dyes, fragrances, or chemicals. Recommended for people with chemical sensitivities and allergies.

- Cruelty-free: No harm was inflicted on animals during the making of the product. The product has not been tested on animals.

- Fair trade: A fair living wage has been guaranteed the (often overseas) workers who manufacture the product. (See more about this in chapter 1.)

- Nontoxic: Contains no toxins that produce harmful effects in people, animals, or the environment when the product is used properly.

- Organic: Ingredients grown and processed according to the USDA's national organic standards, signifying no use of synthetic pesticides, insecticides, herbicides, artificial fertilizers, or genetic engineering.

- Recyclable/reusable: Made from easily recycled materials, or easily reused if not recyclable.

- Socially responsible business: Provides safe and healthy working conditions, fair wages, and respect for their employees.

- Vegan: Contains no animal-derived ingredients.

Bag the Bags!

I went to the store. I bought a wastebasket. The cashier put it in a bag. I brought it home.
I took it out of the bag. I crumpled up the bag and tossed it in the wastebasket.
—LILY TOMLIN

We seem to have gotten away from the old sixties groove of shopping with a collapsible string bag to eliminate wasteful plastic and paper shopping bags. Okay, string bags can be pretty unwieldy, but there are plenty of alternatives. A woman I know back east must have the biggest collection of canvas tote bags in the world. She tosses them into the trunk of her car and pulls them out when she gets to the supermarket or shopping center. Other folks get by with a big backpack. Anything to get away from using plastic bags, which choke municipal drains and wildlife. In Ireland, shopkeepers charge customers for bags. Shopkeepers in India can be fined or shut down for handing out plastic bags. Bangladesh has switched to a traditional and eco-friendly alternative: jute bags. Manufacturers say plastic bags are more hygienic, cheaper to make and buy, and more easily recyclable than paper bags. The trouble is, we don't recycle them all. If you must use bags, choose paper. A paper bag can be reused dozens of times and tossed into the compost pile. But plastic goods may take up to a thousand years to rot. Best of all, do without if you are making a small purchase.

Shop locally first. The best place to spend your dollar is anywhere you can walk, bike, or drive to briefly. Local, independent businesses may provide better advice and service than the larger stores or discount chains. Try to find the nearest natural-foods market or health-food store. They'll carry many of the lesser-known products and brands I refer to in this book.

Troll garage sales, flea markets, junk shops, and antique stores. Places like these are fun to shop at and environmentally benign. The vintage jacket or end table you buy was manufactured ages ago, so it has already made its environmental impact. It'll have no packaging. You'll be supporting a local business. And transporting your find from shop to home will consume less fuel than that set of kitchen knives you snagged on eBay, now wending their way to you from Tokyo.

Use Web and mail-order companies judiciously. How can I possibly badmouth these shopping methods, when they are the only way many of us can bring sensitively made products into our homes? But if you're about to order organic cotton pajamas and duvet covers from across the country, make each shipment count. Wait until you have a sizable order. Consider using retailers that will donate a portion of profits to charity, such as Shop for Change (www.shopforchange.org). Carefully recycle packaging you receive, or bring the materials to a parcel-shipping business near you.

ONE LAST WORD . . .

In the old days people used to window-shop. They'd spend days, months, sometimes years dreaming about a new car, dress, or radio before they ever saved up enough to buy it. It was okay to wander through a department store, looking but not buying. The long waiting period helped people clarify what they were looking for, what mattered most to them. When they finally bought the object of their dreams, they were more likely to treasure it. Sometimes window shopping alone took care of someone's acquisitive longing, and they found they didn't have to buy a thing.

But American culture has changed. We live in a more affluent nation than did our parents and grandparents. Credit and debit cards encourage us to buy things we can't afford. Search engines help us locate collectibles instantly—model trains, books, stamps, glassware—that previously would have taken years to find. That has taken the joy of discovery out of purchases and, in a little way, may contribute to the feeling of emptiness some shoppers feel after they bring their purchases home. Delaying gratification is, ironically, actually a way to make something worth the wait.

CHAPTER 7

PET CARE

No animal should ever jump up on the dining-room furniture
unless absolutely certain that he can hold his own
in the conversation.
—FRAN LEBOWITZ

Not long ago, a large empty television box took center stage on my kitchen floor. The box did not arrive transporting a television, but it did contain lots of theatrics—scratching noises, clucking, and commotion—and provided more entertainment than the Animal Channel. It brought me six baby chickens.

Have you spent any time with a chicken? And before you answer, let me remind you this is not the cooking chapter. Perhaps the domestic chicken is not high on your list of family pets. Golden retriever, black Lab, parakeet, gerbil . . . but chicken?

I've got one word for you: omelets.

I've had enough pets in my lifetime to stock a small petting zoo. Skunks, pigeons, chickens, horses, rabbits, frogs, turtles, hawks, no pigs . . . yet. Oh, and dogs and cats of course. My childhood world was completely intertwined in the animal kingdom—and if any child could talk to animals, I'm sure my sisters and I were steadily on the path of Dr. Doolittle. Pop used to joke that he was the only man around the house, and he had to be careful not to end up neutered like the others.

Those seemingly endless days of crawling eye level with the dogs or trying to train my skunk, Pepé Le Pew, are gone forever. These days what I look for is a sophisticated, independent, and beautiful relationship, and then I consider what pet I want.

Hand-raised chickens are the answer for me: one pair each of White Leghorns, Silver-Laced Wyandottes, and Buff Orpingtons. They have fantastic personalities and show more affection than most cats. They follow me through the garden, eating bugs and providing fertilization in their path. When I pause to inspect a tomato, they often climb aboard my arm or leg and look at me as only an imprinted chicken can. They seem to be saying, "Are you my mother?" In exchange for rearing Winston, Wycliff, Dorothy, Betty-Poop, Einstein, and Mrs. Robinson, I get six organic eggs per day. If I'm going on vacation, my neighbors are happy to help in exchange for the pleasure of fresh eggs.

Raising chickens does impose a few constraints. For starters, you need to check zoning laws. You must also live in a fairly rural area, as house training is out of the question (it's not that chickens aren't smart enough for training, just that they don't have bladders). And you must build a coop that will protect them from their predators, of which there are many. Once you figure out those challenges, you can enjoy all the previously mentioned antics and rewards.

Although I've always loved animals, it was only when I was studying biology in college that I began to see the ways in which humans have affected them. As we saw in the first chapter, indiscriminate use of pesticides, antibiotics, and other chemicals in agriculture can enter the food chain and wreak havoc. Thousands of tiny insects are eaten by one tiny bird, which in turn is consumed by a larger bird of prey. Before long, copious quantities of pesticides either kill the larger animal outright or affect its ability to reproduce. The same thing happens to fish, amphibians, and mammals large and small.

And household pets.

Think about it. Our pets reflect our own health in these inorganic times. A hundred years ago a dog that lived on a farm would have eaten food scraps from its master's table supplemented by whatever it caught in nature. A barn cat's diet was the other way around. But since the food was wholesome, both humans and animals thrived.

The advent of large-scale agribusiness changed all that. Today pets snack on the same pesticide-laden table foods we eat, augmented by commercial pet food that is even worse. The major source of protein found in those bags of dry food or single-serving cans is something the pet industry refers to as the four D's: dead, diseased, disabled, or dying livestock considered unfit for human consumption. When healthy beef, lamb, pork, and chicken do end up in pet food, they're in the form of feathers ("poultry products"), cartilage, tendons, bones, and other "by-products." This method of salvaging discarded fats and proteins and turning it into animal feed has become widely accepted. Burying all this animal waste in a landfill or incinerating it is thought to be disastrous.

Unfortunately, feeding four-D food to our pets and livestock may not be entirely sound. In Europe mad-cow disease was transmitted to new generations of cattle through contaminated feed made from the bodies of their predecessors. In this country, when animals are destroyed at the local pound, their carcasses may be sold to rendering plants and end up in pet food. Many pet companies take pains to ensure that this doesn't happen, but federal law does not prohibit it. A recent study showed some pet food to contain traces of barbiturates—the same ones used to euthanize unwanted pets. Another study found that pet-food companies routinely use discarded restaurant grease as a prime flavoring.

"This is recycling," a spokesperson for the National Renderers' Association said when the grease story broke in the media in 2002. "This process has been used for years. There is no data or study to suggest it isn't safe."

I don't know about you, but that's not my definition of recycling. A number of veterinarians would concur. They're noticing increases in humanlike diseases in pets: diabetes, heart disease, allergies, kidney problems, and cancer. Why is still a matter of opinion. Some vets say that like humans, animals are living longer and are now susceptible to the same ailments we are. That may be true, but while genetics may load the gun, poor nutrition and environmental health pull the trigger. The vets I know insist we cannot ignore the food these animals consume. Our most cherished companions have become the last stop on the human food chain. They get the dregs, and usually they pay a price.

Holistic veterinarian Bob Goldstein and his wife, Susan, learned this firsthand.

SAVING LEIGH

In the 1970s Dr. Bob, a young vet practicing in Westport, Connecticut, where I grew up, adopted a golden retriever named Leigh who suffered from hip dysplasia, a painful genetic ailment common to large dogs. The ligaments in a dysplastic hip are abnormally loose; any energetic movement can throw the hip bone out of its socket, instantly hampering the dog's mobility. Over time the improperly placed bones rub against each other, triggering arthritis and sentencing a dog to a lifetime of pain.

As a pup, Leigh had been selected to train as a Seeing Eye dog, but a year into the program he was rejected because of his poor health. Thinking the pooch would still make a wonderful pet, Dr. Bob and Susan adopted him. His hip problem was going to be a challenge, but after all, Dr. Bob was a vet. He knew what you were supposed to do: administer cortisone to lessen the pain and hope the animal would continue to have a happy life.

> *If a dog jumps into your lap it is because he is fond of you; but if a cat does the same thing it is because your lap is warmer.*
> *—Alfred North Whitehead*

That was the plan, anyway. At the time, Dr. Bob was in his thirties and immersed in a fairly traditional veterinary career. He ran a private practice in town and worked as a researcher at one of the top vet institutions in New York City. He and his colleagues had been trained to use surgery and drugs to treat disease. Anything else just wasn't scientific.

Six years later Dr. Bob and Susan had grown very attached to Leigh. Unfortunately, medicine wasn't working. The dog was still in pain. He whimpered and moaned as he moved slowly around the house. The cortisone injections were beginning to have side effects: Leigh lost muscle mass, his hair thinned in spots, his belly fattened, and he drank water constantly, since the drugs were starting to destroy his kidneys' ability to flush out his system. At age seven, Leigh was going gray in the muzzle. He looked like a dog twice his age.

Dr. Bob surveyed the situation as a medical man would. The next step, he told Susan, was an invasive surgical procedure to rebuild Leigh's hips. If that failed, they'd have to euthanize the dog. There were no other options.

Susan disagreed. Her attitudes toward medicine had been shaped in part by her mom, who died of cancer when Susan was twenty. Susan had devoted her life to helping cancer patients rebuild their strength and immune systems through specialized nutrition. Her work and research focused on alternative medicine and natural healing techniques.

As she listened to her husband lay out their options for Leigh, Susan had a brainstorm. For years she'd been advocating natural foods and vitamin therapy for people. Why couldn't the same work for pets? "It was like a lightbulb went off," she says today. "I told Bob, 'Let's try nutrition first.' "

Leigh's diet changed drastically. The prepared commercial pet food went out the window. Bob and Susan started shopping for him at a health-food market. Leigh ate fresh meats, whole grains, and fibrous vegetables and drank distilled water. Plenty of nights Dr. Bob would come home from work and rev up a juicer to make Leigh some fresh organic carrot juice.

The dog was eating better than they were, and it showed. He looked vibrant. His coat was shiny. Within three weeks Dr. Bob stopped administering cortisone. Leigh's health and mobility continued to improve, and in about ten months he looked like a different dog: he fully regained his mobility, and his coat was a thick, lustrous red-gold color.

Some of the Goldsteins' vet friends poked fun at them. "But you haven't cured anything!" the docs told husband and wife. "His hips are still dysplastic!"

"Who cares?" Susan told 'em. "Look at him! The dog runs, he swims, he fetches! He's leading a normal life."

For Susan it was a vindication of all she'd been saying and studying. For Dr. Bob, the man of science, it was a revelation.

"At the time I was involved in a research project where we were using surgery and chemotherapy for animals with cancer," he recalls. "We'd consider the work a success, but two or three months later the animal would die or have to be put to sleep. I would look at this whole process and think, 'There has to be a better way.'"

His experience with Leigh showed him that there was indeed a better way. But he wasn't about to broadcast it to his colleagues at the research hospital. "In the 1970s there was no way we could even mention this," he says. "There was traditional medicine, and anything outside it was considered quackery. It was clear to me that diet plays a role in healing. I knew I had to introduce this into my practice. So I started offering clients a choice. I'd say, 'We can go the traditional route, or we can try this.'"

It would take ten years of research, but eventually Dr. Bob nailed down a program for natural healing that allows him to treat a host of different pet ailments, such as cancer, arthritis, allergies, and cardiac problems. Veterinary science is very different today than it was when Dr. Bob started out. From four to five thousand vets are holistic practitioners. Dr. Bob now trains other vets in his methods, and Susan edits a national newsletter and runs a successful organic pet-food-and-supply business.

Ironically, caring for pets has changed the way Dr. Bob, Susan, and their two kids eat too. They're passionate about organic foods. Leigh lived to be seventeen years old. That's 119 human years, if you go by the old rule of thumb. We should all be so lucky.

WHAT YOU CAN DO

Here are a few tips that Dr. Bob has shared with me about the care and feeding of your dogs and cats.

Add organic foods or switch to an all-organic diet. This is the best place to start. In your health-food market you'll find organic, natural, or whole-food pet products. These are the best way to be assured that the meat your pet is eating was raised hormone- and drug-free. Under federal law, all pet-food companies must list ingredients on their labels from the greatest to smallest amounts. A label that begins "Beef, beef broth, chicken liver" is infinitely better than one that begins "Beef by-products, water, poultry by-products." With a little practice, you'll begin to spot the whole-food choices. Choose organic supplements to improve fur and skin, clean teeth, and boost the immune system. If this step is too expensive, at the very least start introducing healthier snacks—fresh fruits, vegetables, and grains—into your dog's diet. Read on.

Introduce fresh foods. "No table food!" We've all heard this admonishment for years, but it only makes sense if you and your family eat poorly. As we've seen, the American diet—laden with fats, sugar, and salt and devoid of fiber—is unhealthy for both humans and pets. But if everyone under your roof ate fresh organic fruits, vegetables, meats, and grains, you'd all thrive. In fact, the ideal pet diet would include no commercial pet food. That's too complicated for most people, but what you can do is supplement your pet's organic pet food with healthy fresh foods. For adult dogs and cats, buy a quality pet food intended for *senior* dogs—it has a lower protein content—and add the best chicken, turkey, or beef you can find. This allows you to control the integrity of the protein source. "If someone can't afford this," says Susan Goldstein, "they should do what they can do. Oatmeal's cheap. Brown rice is cheap. Even conventionally grown apples or a cooked potato skin mixed with a good pet food are better than nothing."

Susan suggests the following tips on working fresh treats into your cat or dog's diet. For more advice, see Susan's newsletter, *Love of Animals* (www.earthanimal.com).

Susan uses these "appetite cultivators" to coax stubborn animals to eat new, healthful fare. (Buy organic whenever possible.)

FLAVOR ENHANCERS

Grated cheese (feta or Swiss)

Low-fat plain yogurt

Beef and chicken broth

Eggs (poached, or hard-boiled and chopped)

Cottage cheese (low-fat, low-sodium)

Nut milks (1 cup of almonds or cashews blended with 1 cup
filtered water)

FAVORITE FAST SNACKS

Apples, chopped and cored

Pears, chopped

Melon balls

Grapes (must be organic)

Bananas (must be organic)

Applesauce (must be organic)

Oatios (fruit-juice-sweetened oat rings found at health-food
stores)

Brussels sprouts

Zucchini sticks

Whole carrots

Popcorn (homemade, unbuttered, unsalted)

Shredded wheat (sugar-free)

Matzoh (whole-wheat)

Brown-rice crackling cereal (health-food version)

THE BEST BASIC JUICE

Freshly juiced organic carrots make a superb drink. If your animal doesn't care for the taste straight up, mix with freshly juiced apples or celery, or add directly to drinking water. Serve cats and small dogs (up to 25 pounds) a quarter of a cup; larger dogs one cup.

FOODS TO AVOID

White refined flour	Fish or chicken with bones
Refined sugar	Meat fat or chicken fat
Iodized salt	Citrus
Pork	Tomatoes
Bacon and cured meats	Candy, chocolate, or sweets of
Organ meat unless organic	any kind

Keep air fresh and water clean. Your pets are just as vulnerable as you are to polluted indoor air and chlorinated tap water. Offer your pet the same water you filter for your family, and open the windows now and then. If you are concerned about airborne pollutants such as bacteria, gases, pollen, dander, mold, fungi, or smoke, consider an air purifier for heavily used rooms in your home.

Petproof your home. Curious about their environments, pets will investigate, mouth, and tussle with almost any item in your home. Here are ways to keep them safe.

- Hide electrical cords or wipe them with cayenne pepper and olive oil, which will ward off any curious puppy or kitten. Similarly, tie up the cords on venetian blinds. Give your pets plenty of toys to play with so they don't seek amusement elsewhere.

- Use stainless steel or sealed ceramic bowls. Beside being chewable, plastic bowls (and toys, for that matter) emit gases left over from the manufacturing process that can irritate your pet's nose or leach into food.

- Choose house and garden plants carefully. Common houseplants such as poinsettia, dieffenbachia, and mistletoe are highly toxic. Outdoors, beautiful flowering plants such as foxglove, larkspur, and lupine likewise pose threats to children and pets. It's best to buy plants and seeds from reputable nurseries, where salespeople can advise you on the toxicity of a plant before you buy. To keep pets away from the plants you do have,

Susan Goldstein recommends planting alfalfa sprouts and keeping a tempting tray of them where your pet can reach it.

- Watch the heavy machinery. Animals have a habit of sneaking into unlikely places for naps. Close the doors to washers and dryers. Ask a mechanic to screen off the fan-belt area in your car engine. Disconnect power tools. And close off air vents and openings leading to major appliances.

Eliminate cigarette smoke. No surprise here: secondhand smoke imperils adults, children, and pets alike.

Learn animal first aid. Ask your veterinarian for information on how to care for your pet in an emergency. Keep the poison-control phone number next to your phone. Practice pet CPR and mouth-to-mouth resuscitation.

- Selling commercial pet food is an $11 billion-a-year industry in the United States.

- Ninety percent of vets surveyed say they worry about the quality of commercial pet food.

- Cancer is the number one disease that kills cats and dogs in the United States.

- Twenty-five percent of all animal-shelter pets are purebred. In seven years, a fertile cat and her offspring can theoretically produce 420,000 kittens.

(Sources: Morris Animal Foundation, Animal Protection Institute, Humane Society)

Skip the household poisons and pesticides. The American home is chock-full of dangerous toxins that imperil adults, children, and pets. Your pets are especially vulnerable; like small children, they spend their entire lives close to the ground, sniffing and licking surfaces an adult human wouldn't dare touch. Indoors, they're easy prey for residues from toilet cleaners, furniture polish, and floor waxes. Newly installed synthetic carpets and most carpet cleaners are highly toxic. Outdoors, pets can inhale or ingest harmful lawn-care products, pest sprays, and car-wash water. In the garage they may be tempted by the syrupy smell and taste of antifreeze. Consider switching to less toxic items, or lock up the ones you have. When you hire exterminators, pool specialists, and landscapers, ask them to use biodegradable, harmless preparations to get their jobs done. (We'll tell you more about that in the next chapter.)

Look for natural, organic pest repellents, soaps, and shampoos. Carefully choose the products you apply directly to your animal's body. You'll find alternatives to toxic flea-and-tick collars and shampoos at your health-food store. (Dr. Bob once cooked up a pet shampoo so mild he uses it still to wash his own hair.) A good diet can also help your pet naturally repel irritating or dangerous pests. Herbal remedies are also effective, but before you mix your own, consult with a holistic veterinarian.

Choose a holistic veterinarian. Bet you saw this one coming a mile away. Veterinary medicine has come a long way since the 1970s when Dr. Bob adopted Leigh. These days vets are likely to be more progressive than their human-treating colleagues. It's quite easy to find a vet who stays current in both conventional medicine and alternative therapies such as natural healing, enhanced nutrition, acupuncture, and homeopathy. You can get information and locate vets near you through the American Holistic Veterinary Medical Association (www.ahvma.org) and Alt Vet Med (www.altvetmed.com).

Test blood, hold off on vaccines. A growing number of vets believe that our animals are being overvaccinated. We would not give a child shots every year, they argue, but we routinely do this with animals. In some cases pets have developed skin tumors near the vaccination sites. Before you schedule booster shots, consider having the animal's blood tested to investigate the efficacy of previous shots. A powerful diagnostic tool, a blood analysis can also reveal illness before it strikes, or nutritional deficiencies to help you plan the animal's diet. If your vet is unsure how to do this, ask him or her to contact Dr. Bob's testing firm, BioNutritional Diagnostics (www.bnaweb.com).

For more information on pet diseases, care, political issues, and resources for locating vets in your area, see the Resources Directory.

One Last Word . . .

I'd be remiss if I didn't point out that there is an excellent environmental argument for *not* having pets. Simply put, the more mouths we have to feed on the face of the earth, the more resources we must consume to do it. Each year the number of humans and their menagerie of domestic animals grows. Farm animals. Working animals. Performing animals. Research animals. And the list goes on. By one estimate, humans, our livestock, and our pets comprise 80 percent of the mass of the world's vertebrates. Wild animals account for the rest. The stories about animals being rendered and ending up in pet food are indeed appalling, but that carnage could be abated if we humans chose to eat lower on the food chain and breed fewer pets. I know that's easier said than done.

I grew up loving animals, and my respect for science and the earth was born out of caring for these creatures. When I hear that each year eight to ten million animals are surrendered to shelters and four or five million, conservatively, are euthanized, I wonder what can be done. One option is to love the animals we have before breeding more. If you and your kids want a pet, there's no better place to look for one than a shelter. All my family's pets have come from shelters, and what an amusing menagerie they've been. If you like animals but aren't sure if you can care for one long-term, please don't adopt any. Instead, support the good work of wildlife organizations and animal sanctuaries.

The days are gone when I kept loads of pets. I keep my chickens, give them feed, and in return they eat insects and drop plenty of manure I'll toss on my garden someday. Whenever I see them clucking around the yard, I am again reminded of the natural cycle I share with them and the earth. I wouldn't give that up for the world. Besides, I need the eggs.

CHAPTER 8

CLEANING AND HOUSEHOLD PESTS

There was no need to do any housework after all.
After the first four years the dirt
doesn't get any worse.
—QUENTIN CRISP

I visited some Anasazi ruins in Arizona a few years back. These beautiful dwellings were home to indigenous peoples for hundreds of years. Still evident was the cliff-dwelling dump site—a small pile of bird bones and corn husks. How natural, I thought. How beautiful these dwellings nestle into the landscape. How tidy things look—even after six hundred years! Is my home so different because I have hardwood flooring? Did the Anasazi have ant problems?

A pest is something that annoys us. Annoying doesn't mean not useful, so "pest" is a relative term. Consider stoplights. Annoying? Sometimes. Essential? Probably. It is safe to say I like my ants, rats, mice, and wasps on the outside of my house, doing what they've been doing for hundreds of millions of their generations (compared with us, we who have existed a piddly hundred thousand generations). And I like my stoplights green.

That said, I realize our cultural evolution has greatly accelerated change in nature over the past few centuries, exceeding the rate of organic evolution by orders of magnitude. We all know the cockroaches will outlive humanity—just ask anyone who lives in New York City. Yet we try to obliterate vast numbers of "pests" in our world—often with far-reaching consequences—rendering our biosphere a far less beautiful and interesting place to occupy.

Our culture is selective—dandelions are weeds, ants spoil picnics, mosquitoes ruin a camping trip. Okay, so maybe mosquitoes should go—but the key here seems to be a little respect, even for the creepy crawly creature that we don't want in our backyard. Somewhere this creature has a place in our ecosystem, and just because we don't understand its place during this particular picnic doesn't mean this "pest" shouldn't serve as a reminder of what a wonderful and diverse planet this was before we started cutting up the watermelon.

My home and all the domestic activities within are nothing more than a reflection of the larger world. It is so easy to ignore the source of the energy and water arriving to the house and the soap and garbage leaving. It is far too easy to spray that weed killer, use a little more bleach on that coffee stain, and poison those rats. But when does it stop? When do we realize there is no separation between our homes and the ecosystem? We are nature—and although our homes look very different from Anasazi ruins, it's all relative to what our homes will look like in the year 2080.

I've come to enjoy the extra responsibility that accompanies knowledge about our interconnected environment. It is really about self-respect, for if not us, then who? If not now, when? Besides, I really don't want future humans to be sporting an exoskeleton.

One of my favorite lectures from college was on the second law of thermodynamics: everything moves from a state of order to disorder. Actually, I only really understand it as far as it relates to my house, which gets dirty even when I'm away on vacation (I think the wind in cliff dwellings may be marketable). And speaking of college science class, one of my favorite authors is E. O. Wilson, who writes beautifully on, among other topics, the field of myrmecology, the study of ants: how they make war, reproduce, bury their dead, and use propaganda and surveillance. For an adult homeowner, however, ants, with their wonderful miniature yet immense civilization, are a completely different study. I don't appreciate them in my kitchen and have nothing short of a war going on each winter.

With all due respect for ants and Sir Isaac Newton, I'd like to offer a few stories and tools to help you live as gracefully as possible while respecting the principle of least impact with greatest results. Richard Cooper is a great example of someone who does just that.

BUGGED BY A CLIENT: INTEGRATED PEST MANAGEMENT

A bakery owner had a problem. His kitchen was overrun with about a hundred yellow-jacket wasps, which were buzzing and hovering over his workers as they cranked out their baker's dozens. The owner called Cooper Pest Control, near Princeton, New Jersey. Richard Cooper, who runs the company with his brother Phil, answered the call.

Rick is not your ordinary pesticide-toting technician. He kind of likes bugs. He spent his boyhood collecting them, his college years studying them, and his adult years breeding some in his company's office (in terrariums and test tubes, of course). Whenever he visits schools to talk about bugs, he takes along his giant Madagascar hissing cockroaches and African millipedes. Like any entomologist, he knows that every critter has special habits. If you know what makes them tick, you can outwit them and keep them out of your home.

That is part of the new philosophy embraced by many modern American pest-control companies. For decades, exterminators were little more than hired guns summoned to do a single job: kill bugs dead. Pesticides were the cornerstone of the pest-control industry, and were applied routinely to control a wide variety of pests. What rodents or bugs they didn't kill often lived to sire toxin-resistant descendants. To wipe out ensuing generations, scientists were obliged to cook up more and more dangerous chemicals. That approach can't last forever, and exterminators know it. These days the best pest-control companies practice "integrated pest management" (IPM), a technique that minimizes the use of pesticides and challenges technicians to ask the bigger question—why and how are pests getting in? IPM technicians work from the least toxic solution on up: prevention, trapping, and finally pesticides with minimal toxicity.

When Rick Cooper got to the bakery that day, his brain was thinking like a yellow jacket's. He knew the brightly colored wasps love sugary liquids. Sure enough, in the backyard of the bakery were some dirty bakers' trays—all of them oozing jams, jellies, and frostings—and a Dumpster. It was a hot August day, and the staff had propped open the back door. The yellow jackets had been partying around the Dumpster, and inevitably some had migrated indoors.

> For the first time in the history of the world, every human being is now subjected to contact with dangerous chemicals, from the moment of conception until death.
> —*Rachel Carson*, Silent Spring (1962)

Rick rattled off a bunch of recommendations to the owner. Clean up your act. Wash down the trays and outdoor area with a power hose. Move the Dumpster away from the facility. Install air conditioning. And keep the back door shut. The angry baker shot down every idea. "The Dumpster stays! I don't have any space back here to move it. And air conditioning's too expensive."

"Well, can you at least put in a screen door?"

"I suppose so. But look, you still have to bomb this place! I can't have these yellow jackets flying around!"

Rick couldn't believe what he was hearing. The guy wanted him to fog the kitchen. "I can't do that," Rick told him. "It's illegal to do that while you're open and food is exposed."

"Look," the baker told him, "either you do it, or I'll just go to the hardware store, get some stuff, and do it myself."

(He could do just that. In recent years organophosphates—the same chemical family that includes DDT—have been banned from professional use. But ironically, homeowners can still walk into a hardware store, buy 'em, and misapply 'em.) But Rick knew he could take care of the situation. Armed with the knowledge that yellow jackets love light, he went into the kitchen, shut the doors, killed the lights, and used aprons to cover all but one window, which he left open a crack. In less than a minute, every yellow jacket zipped to the well-lighted window and flew away.

Mission accomplished.

Of course, the baker didn't see it that way. A few days later, he called Rick back, and he was seeing red. Or rather, yellow.

"I'm not paying your bill!" the guy griped. "You didn't apply anything, and all those wasps are all back inside the kitchen!"

I applied knowledge, Rick thought to himself. "Why are they back?" he asked the baker. "Did you move the Dumpster away from your building like I recommended?"

"No!"

"Did you clean up the area outside your restaurant? Did you install a screen door?"

"No! Look, are you gonna come spray, or do I have to call someone else?"

The guy was pretty thickheaded. He wanted pesticides outside his kitchen, where he cooked and served food to his customers. And yet, if he only modified his habits, the wasps would lose interest and split. Pests are nothing but opportunistic. If they can't find food or a way in, they'll move on.

Sometimes the customers do too. The baker hung up and never called back. Rick surmises the guy found an exterminator who would do what he wanted: kill those bugs dead.

He never did pay that darn bill.

I suppose trailblazers like Rick know they risk being misunderstood, even mocked. Mark Twain said, "The man with the new idea is a crank until the idea succeeds." Certainly Emanuel Bronner suffered his share of indignities before he earned everyone's respect.

A Clean Break with the Past

They called him the pope of soap, the sultan of suds. He longed to unite humankind but spent years estranged from his own family. Some people thought him mad, others saw him as a commercial genius. His name was Emanuel Bronner, and he was a little bit of both.

Born to the Heilbrunner family of German soap makers, Bronner emigrated as a young man to the United States in 1929. As a boy studying his craft, he had learned that true soap is absolutely natural, a by-product of a chemical reaction between lye and fats such as vegetable oils or animal tallow. His Orthodox Jewish father made ultramild castile soap, using olive oil as the prime ingredient. Bronner's dad was a tough cookie. In fact, the family still laughs when recalling that when Bronner tried to organize his father's workers, the old man bought him a one-way ticket to America. Once here, the young man changed his name and prowled the Midwest, working a string of consulting jobs for American soap companies. Bronner saw that Americans were losing interest in finely crafted soaps and cleaners. The goal was mass production, and to reach that goal, the oil-rich nation was experimenting with petroleum-based products instead.

In the years following World War II, radio and TV commercials lobbed a host of soaps, detergents, and cleansers at the American public. These products, originally designed for industrial purposes, were better suited to swabbing down an oil rig than human skin, clothes, and furnishings, but they were plentiful and convenient, and Americans snapped them off the shelves.

By the war's end, Bronner had lost his young wife to illness and his parents to the Nazis. Racked with grief, guilt, and disillusionment, he dreamed of a world united under one God and a common goal: peace. When not working he gave peace talks and distributed leaflets. His eccentricity branded him a troublemaker, and after a series of bizarre incidents, one of his sisters had him committed to an Illinois mental institution, where he was subjected to electroshock treatments that would haunt him for the rest of his life. While he languished inside, his three children ended up in a string of foster homes. After three attempts, he escaped the hospital. Now a fugitive, he scrounged up some cash, bid farewell to his kids, and hightailed it to California.

His salvation, of course, lay in soap. In a dingy Los Angeles hotel room in 1946 he began mixing batches of his family recipe, and soon he was selling bottles of Dr. Bronner's Magic Soaps in health-food stores.

From the start, his labels were, well, a little peculiar. Bronner's instructions for using his liquid soap read: "Warning! Keep Out of Eyes! Wash Out with Water! Don't Drink Soap! Dilute! Dilute! Or Wet Skin Well! OK!" Elsewhere on the bottle he printed his rambling philosophies for saving "Spaceship Earth," uniting the world's peoples, and staying healthy and clean. A typical bottle might include as many as three thousand words in minuscule, eye-straining type. He quoted the Torah, the Koran, the Bible. He shared the words of Christ, Confucius, the Buddha, Mohammed, Gandhi, and Einstein. He railed against Communists and Nazis. And he offered up his own "Moral ABCs." At times these pithy maxims were, like Bronner's own speech, hard to follow. Customers didn't so much read them as they read between the lines.

1ˢᵗ: Absolute cleanliness is Godliness!
2ⁿᵈ: Constructive-selfish hard work save home-food-young!
3ʳᵈ: Absolute teamwork fertilizes God's earth!

Smile, help teach the whole Human race,
the Moral ABC of All-One-God-Faith,
Lightning-like Strong & we're All-One!
All-One!

It took some time, but eventually the strange soaps were embraced by the American counterculture. When Bronner was reunited with his sons in the mid-fifties, he put them to work, Ralph typing labels and sending out invoices, Jim as a chemist. The kids were stunned to see that their old man's soap was catching on.

And with good reason. After washing with Dr. Bronner's, your skin felt as clean and soft as a baby's. There was no residue on your skin or tub. Habitués of health-food stores liked the soap's all-natural ingredients. Bikers loved the way it cut grease and used it to wash their choppers. Park rangers and wilderness guides recommended it to campers, grateful that the soap didn't pollute streams and rivers. And sixties flower children found that life on the commune was infinitely more bearable when you had a quart of Dr. Bronner's all-purpose soap around.

What About Dry Cleaning?

Dry cleaning is anything but dry. The clothes you drop off are doused with perchloroethylene, "perc" for short, a chemical solvent that has been linked to liver cancer. If you like to have your clothes professionally cleaned and don't want to go the wash, starch, and press route yourself, look for a "wet cleaner" near you. These greener companies use either delicate soaps to launder fine washables or recyclable liquid carbon dioxide (CO_2). To find a suitable wet cleaner near you, see the Professional Wetcleaning Network's website (www.tpwn.net).

When Bronner started making his soaps in the forties, there was no such thing as an environmental movement. But times have changed. Now Americans are acutely aware that something is not right in our air, water, and soil. The EPA says the air in the average home is far more dangerous than outdoor air. And the American College of Allergists says 50 percent of all illnesses can be traced back to home sweet home. The source of all these ills are the toxic cleaners and pesticides lurking in cabinets and closets. Every toxin used around the home goes down the drain or into a landfill, where it stands a chance of leaching back into drinking water.

Public-works officials, water companies, and sewage authorities are beginning to encourage citizens to use less toxic detergents and cleaners. A number of small companies are making soaps and cleaners the old-fashioned way, out of biodegradable substances. Over the Internet and through university co-op extension offices, environmentally conscious Americans are also swapping recipes for homemade household cleaners. If you scan those lists, you're sure to find a familiar ingredient amid the baking soda, vinegar, and lemon juice: Dr. Bronner's Magic Soaps.

Bronner was clearly ahead of his time. Today, when you walk the aisles of a health-food store, organic market, or even some big conventional supermarkets, you'll find biodegradable soaps, detergents, dishwashing liquids, and other products that go easy on the earth.

> *Man does not live by soap alone.*
> —*G. K. Chesterton*

WHO LET THE (WATCH)DOG OUT?
THE FALLACY OF CHEMICAL-SAFETY STANDARDS

Since the end of World War II, seventy to eighty thousand chemicals have been released in the environment through new consumer and industrial products and food. "Most Americans would assume that basic toxicity testing is available and that all chemicals in commerce today are safe," reads a report from the EPA's Office of Pollution Prevention and Toxics. "A recent EPA study has found that this is not a prudent assumption." According to the EPA's report:

- The United States produces or imports close to three thousand chemicals at over one million pounds per year per chemical. The EPA has reviewed the publicly available data on these chemicals and has found that most may have never been tested to determine how toxic they are to humans or the environment.

- International authorities agree that six basic tests are necessary for a minimum understanding of a chemical's toxicity. Of these three thousand high-production-volume chemicals, 93 percent are missing one or more of these basic tests; 43 percent are missing *all* of them. Only 7 percent of these chemicals have undergone all six of the most basic screening tests.

Are Kids at Risk?

You won't find a single toxic cleaner in Elizabeth Sword's house. Some years ago, when she became interested in children's environmental health, she began seriously reading labels on the products in her home and created an ambitious program to eliminate toxins. Today, she tells us, she swears by baking soda and vinegar and the occasional sprinkle of borax.

By no coincidence, she's president of a group called the Children's Health Environmental Coalition (CHEC), which has helped bring attention to the impact of dangerous products on children's health. The group has noted a disturbing trend: rates of asthma, learning disabilities, and cancer in children are all up over the last twenty years. The number of cancer cases among American children younger than fifteen has been steadily rising at the rate of nearly 1 percent per year. Leukemia and brain tumors account for the biggest leaps.

Now, science is far from being able to link these increases to the proliferation of household chemicals. But I think it doesn't hurt to play it safe. Kids live their lives close to the ground, where traces of household chemicals inevitably deposit. Their growing bodies more readily absorb chemicals than the bodies of adults. And children more often touch surfaces indiscriminately or stick objects in their mouths. Their unborn siblings can also be affected by toxins, even while in the womb.

"There are things people can do right now, tonight, to keep their homes safe," says Elizabeth, a mother of three. "You can take your shoes off when you come home. That costs nothing. You can open the windows more often. You can stop using toxic cleaners. If you see an ant in the kitchen, instead of reaching for a spray can, you can start to ask yourself, 'Well, why is he there?' Everything you do will be an automatic plus for your family." CHEC's website (www.checnet.org) features a handy diagnostic tool, "Health-e-Home," that walks browsers through common household toxins and where they lurk in the home.

Plants That Clean Air

B. C. Wolverton is a chemist who pioneered the use of house and office plants to eliminate airborne toxins. He designed his own home in Picayune, Mississippi, to exploit the air-scrubbing properties of plants. In his beautifully illustrated book, *How to Grow Fresh Air* (Penguin, 1997), Dr. Wolverton recommends fifty plants that clean air best. For more information, see his website (www.wolvertonenvironmental.com). In the botanical world, these top ten houseplants are just what the doctor ordered:

Areca palm (*Chrysalidocarpus lutescens*)
Lady palm (*Rhapis excelsa*)
Bamboo palm (*Chamaedorea seifrizii*)
Rubber plant (*Ficus robusta*)
Dracaena "Janet Craig" (*Dracaena deremensis* "Janet Craig")
English ivy (*Hedera helix*)
Dwarf date palm (*Phoenix roebelenii*)
Ficus alii (*Ficus macleildandii* "Alii")
Boston fern (*Nephrolepsis exaltata* "*Bostoniensis*")
Peace lily (*Spathiphyllum sp.*)

WHAT YOU CAN DO

Here are some ways to clean your home and get rid of pests that won't come back to haunt you. Your place will look good and smell great. Like farmers who reap organic crops, you too can be a steward of the earth, land, and water.

Take an inventory of all the toxic products in your home.

- Take time to empty the cabinets and shelves in your kitchen, bathrooms, laundry room, garage, and shed. Look for pesticides and cleaning materials, along with empty paint cans, solvents, automobile fluids, wood-finishing products, and flammable liquids.

- Study the labels to gauge the relative danger posed to you, your family, or your pets by keeping this stuff around. Decide whether you can live with it, slowly using it up, or would like to dispose of it in an ecologically sound manner. You may have spent a wad of cash on laundry detergents or cleaning products. As you use them up, keep an eye out for less toxic alternatives. (See the "Reading Labels" sidebar.)

Reading Labels

By law, household products must be labeled according to their level of immediate toxicity. Here's what those labels mean:

Caution: Least toxic. Lethal dose is 1 ounce to 1 pint.

Warning: Toxic. Lethal dose is 1 teaspoon to 1 tablespoon.

Danger (or *Poison*): Most toxic. Lethal dose is 1 taste to 1 teaspoon.

The EPA recognizes four attributes of hazardous substances:

Toxic: Toxic materials (such as pesticides, weed killers, and many household cleaners) can poison people and pets. Toxic substances can cause illness and even death if swallowed or absorbed through the skin.

Corrosive: Corrosive products (such as drain, oven, and acid-based toilet cleaners) can severely burn skin and eyes, or internal organs if swallowed.

Ignitable: Ignitable products (such as kerosene, paint and furniture-polish solvents, and spot removers) will catch fire if heated or placed near a flame.

Reactive: Reactive materials can explode or create poisonous gas when combined with other chemicals. (Chlorine bleach and ammonia create a poisonous gas when mixed.)

- If you choose to dispose of this stuff, call your local sanitation department and ask if they will accept any of it. In some communities, hazardous-waste collection is conducted on the county level only on selected days. Be patient as you phone around. The information you glean from these calls will enable you to plan future purchases. If there's some product that your town or county cannot properly dispose of, consider discontinuing use of that product.

Replace what you've discarded with store-bought, earth-friendly products. Here's a list to get you started. It is hardly encyclopedic. The next time you need a cleaning product, consider visiting a health-food store to see what products they stock. Scrutinize the labels carefully. Reputable companies will list all ingredients on the packaging; some also state how many days it takes for their product to break down in the environment.

- Two well-known brands of soaps, cleaners, and detergents—Seventh Generation (www.seventhgen.com) and Ecover (www.ecover.com)—are widely available at health-food stores. Retail websites offer information on brands such as Bio-Kleen (www.biokleen.com), Orange-Glo (www.greatcleaners.com), and Citra-Solv (www.shadowlake.com). "Old-fashioned" cleaners also make safer alternatives. Murphy's Vegetable Oil Soap (www.murphyoilsoap.com) is biodegradable and phosphate-free. Bon Ami (www.faultless.com) is a mild, chlorine-free abrasive made with feldspar, a naturally occurring mineral.

- Just because a product is organic or less toxic doesn't mean it won't harm you if swallowed or splashed on skin and eyes. Observe the usual precautions, and try to use as little as you need to get the job done.

- Can't find it? Search the list of vendors at Coop America (www.coopamerica.org) or EcoCities (www.ecocities.net/Shopping.htm).

Replace conventional cleaning products with homemade cleaners. Making your own cleaning products is cheaper than buying conventional and green cleaners. A quart of distilled white vinegar—a potent household-grease cutter—costs about fifty cents, compared with two to four dollars for a quart of store-bought cleaners. This option will offset other expenses and reduce consumption of plastic bottles and cardboard boxes. Sponges, a few brushes, a funnel, rubber gloves, a couple of good spray bottles, and a bucket are all the "hardware" you need. Use an old teaspoon to sprinkle baking soda out of the box. Reuse old spray bottles to dispense vinegar or other liquid cleaners, but wash the bottle well first. If you have a need that isn't covered here, search online for nontoxic homemade household cleaners.

The Worst Offenders

Here's just a partial list of some of the chemicals found in many household products and their effects. Unfortunately, they may or may not be listed on the packaging. Manufacturers are required to list all "active" ingredients considered immediate hazards. Inert ingredients—extra compounds that "carry" the active ingredient to do its job—don't have to be listed but may have long-term effects. Check the list of ingredients before you buy.

Air Fresheners
Formaldehyde: Highly toxic. Suspected carcinogen.
Phenol: Causes skin to swell, burn, peel, and break out in hives.
Paradichlorobenzene: Dangerous to internal organs if inhaled, to skin with prolonged exposure. Causes nausea, vomiting, diarrhea, liver and kidney damage if ingested.

Ammonia
Volatile chemical, very damaging to eyes, respiratory tract, and skin. Repeated or prolonged exposure may cause irritation, bronchitis, and pneumonia.

Antibacterial Cleaners
Triclosan: Linked to liver damage.

Antifreeze
Ethylene glycol: Very toxic; 3 ounces can be fatal to adults. Damages cardiovascular systems, blood, skin, and kidneys.
Methanol: Moderately toxic; ingestion may cause coma, respiratory damage.

Carpet and Upholstery Shampoos

Perchlorethylene: Suspected carcinogen; causes liver, kidney, and nervous-system damage.

Ammonium hydroxide: Corrosive, extremely irritable to eyes, skin, and respiratory passages.

Car Waxes, Polishes

Petroleum distillates: Linked to skin and lung cancer; irritates skin, eyes, nose, lungs. Can cause fatal pulmonary edema if inhaled.

Chlorine Bleach

Sodium hypochlorite: Strongly corrosive. Irritates or burns skin, eyes, and respiratory tract. May cause pulmonary edema or vomiting and coma if ingested.

Dishwasher Detergents

May contain chlorine in a dry form.

Disinfectants

Sodium hypochlorite (as in chlorine bleach).

Phenols (as in air fresheners).

Drain Cleaners

Sodium or potassium hydroxide (lye): Caustic, burns skin and eyes; if ingested will damage esophagus and stomach.

Hydrochloric acid: Corrosive, eye and skin irritant, damages kidneys, liver, and digestive tract.

Trichloromethane: Eye and skin irritant, nervous-system depressant; damages liver and kidneys.

Flea Powders

Carbaryl: Very toxic, interferes with human nervous system; can cause skin, respiratory, and cardiovascular damage.

Dichlorophene: Skin irritant. Can damage liver, kidney, spleen, and central nervous system.

Floor Cleaners/Waxes

Diethylene glycol: Can cause central nervous-system depression and kidney, liver lesions.

Petroleum solvents: Flammable. Linked to skin and lung cancer. Irritates skin, eyes, nose, throat, and lungs.

Furniture Polishes

Petroleum distillates (as in car waxes and polishes).

Phenol (as in air fresheners).

Nitrobenzene: Easily absorbed through the skin; extremely toxic.

Laundry-Room Products

Sodium or calcium hypochlorite (as in chlorine bleach).

Linear alkylate sulfonate: Absorbed through the skin. Known liver-damaging agent.

Sodium tripolyphosphate: Irritates skin and mucous membranes, causes vomiting. Easily absorbed through the skin from clothes.

Mold-and-Mildew Cleaners

Sodium hypochlorite (as in chlorine bleach).

Formaldehyde (as in air fresheners).

Oven Cleaners

Sodium hydroxide (lye) (as in drain cleaners).

Toilet-Bowl Cleaners

Hydrochloric acid: Highly corrosive; irritant to both skin and eyes. Damages kidneys and liver.

Sodium hypochlorite (as in chlorine bleach).

- **All-purpose cleaner.** Fill a spray bottle with half water, half distilled white vinegar; add a spoonful of biodegradable liquid soap.

- **Bathroom surfaces.** Moisten the surface, scrub with baking soda or a chlorine- or ammonia-free cleanser such as Bon Ami. Between cleanings, scrub toilets lightly with a moistened brush. Old toothbrushes are perfect for hard-to-reach spots.

- **Carpet cleaner.** Blot fresh stains with club soda. Or sprinkle cornstarch and vacuum for general cleaning. Apply a baking-soda paste, then vacuum.

- **Disinfecting.** Clean surface with our 50/50 vinegar-water solution. Or try ½ cup of borax dissolved in a gallon of hot water, scented with fresh lemon juice. Dry well, since germs thrive in moisture.

- **Drain cleaner.** Sprinkle ½ cup of baking soda down the drain, followed by ½ cup of vinegar. (Do not do this if the drain has recently been cleaned with chlorine or a chlorine-based product. It can cause dangerous fumes.) Then pour boiling water down the drain. To prevent reclogging, cover the drain with a filter to keep out hair and food particles.

- **Oven cleaner.** While the oven is still warm, apply baking soda (or salt) with a damp sponge. Let dry, then scour with fine-grade, soapless steel wool.

- **Pots and pans.** Drain all liquid grease from the pan into a spare container. Sprinkle on baking soda, scrub, and rinse. For baked crud, moisten the pan, sprinkle on the soda, and let it soften.

- **Windows and mirrors.** Use the 50/50 water-vinegar spray. Wipe with a lint-free cloth (like an old diaper) instead of paper towels, which leave dust behind (and waste trees).

Chemicals You Should Never Mix

Never mix chlorine bleach with ammonia (or vinegar). The result of these reactions is chloramine gas, which is highly irritating to lungs and causes coughing and choking.

Rock Star

Peter is the Newman's Own Organics CCBW (chief cook and bottle washer). But in his own home, he's chief tile-and-toilet scrubber. (His wife handles the checkbook.) Peter swears by pumice. He uses one of those little stones to "erase" tough mineral deposits on porcelain, tile, and grout. Buff, buff, buff, and the stuff's gone. "It won't harm porcelain or tile," he says, "but you wouldn't want to do it on stainless steel or any other metal." Peter's so enamored of this tip, he's shared it with quite a few folks around the office. It works so well that he's got some groupies.

Practice Green Pest Control

- In many cases, you can end a pest problem by cleaning the infested area and removing the food source. If you insist on buying pest-control products, confine yourself to ones labeled "Caution."

- Use "homemade" or "natural" pesticide remedies with caution. Cayenne pepper, garlic sprays, and other herbal approaches can do harm if misused or overapplied. "I've done experiments with hot pepper oil that have burned my eyes and nasal passages," says Rick Cooper. "I've been afraid to let children and pets outside after I've sprayed." "Natural" does not necessarily mean safe.

- If the infestation continues unabated, call in an IPM professional. "Look for someone who takes a holistic approach, and interview them," says Rick Cooper. "What's their philosophy? Are they solving problems, or just spraying? If they say, 'We'll come out and spray,' you know what you're dealing with."

- If it comes down to a pesticide application, ask the technician to explain your options—from the least toxic preparations up.

- Stay informed. See the Beyond Pesticides (www.beyondpesticides.org) or the Bio-Integral Resource Center (www.birc.org) websites to locate a pro in your area.

A Pest-Control Sampler

The following are a mix of common-sense tips and a few natural remedies. Homemade approaches don't work for everyone, and scientific evidence supporting them is sparse. If something proves ineffective—even if it works for someone else—discontinue its use.

Ants. Ants travel along chemical trails left by their platoon leader. Obliterate all evidence of previous invasions by wiping down counters and floors with a vinegar-and-water solution and removing the alluring food or water. If the problem persists, hire a pro to seal them out of your home.

Fleas. Look for herbal flea collars at your health-food store. They contain plant-based oils that repel fleas, such as pennyroyal, eucalyptus, and citronella. You can also give your animal a bath, and then rub these same oils (available at a health-food store) through their coats. (Pennyroyal, a kind of mint oil, should not be used around pregnant women or animals.) Some pet owners experience good results with garlic-yeast tablets, available through pet stores. If you need to stop an outbreak immediately, choose flea treatments whose active ingredients are citrus-based (d-limonene) or herb-based (erigeron and rose geranium). During flea season, clean your home frequently, and take time to launder your animal's bedding.

Grain pests. Store bulk grains, flours, spices, and other dry pantry foods for no longer than three months. Keep in airtight glass, hard plastic, or tin containers. Plastic freezer bags don't work, as determined pests can chew right through them. Tupperware is good, but you must activate the seal.

Moths. Before you store clothes for the season, have them cleaned, or air them in bright sunlight and brush well with a stiff brush. Moth larvae feed on food stains, dried sweat, and other residues, and dislodge easily from fabric. Try storing clothes with cedar chips or sprigs of dried lavender flowers to repel adult moths.

Patio insects. Burn citronella candles and apply a DEET-free insect repellant to your skin. Skip bug zappers, as they kill beneficial bugs along with the bad.

Roaches. Again, scrupulously clean the area and eliminate food sources. Boric acid is a natural time-honored roach killer and simple to use. Roaches are famously resilient, and you may need to hire help to deal with a persistent problem.

Rodents. Clean areas under stoves, refrigerators, and dishwashers. Store dry human and pet food in airtight containers. Clean pet bowls each night. Place wild-bird feeders away from your house. Use tight-fitting lids on thick plastic or metal trash cans. Keep garage doors closed.

- If these measures don't work, move on to snap traps. On your first outing, bait the traps but don't set them. You want to train mice to expect easy food. Later, place baited traps in the areas of the house where you suspect activity, but be sure you can reach the trap afterward. The trap goes perpendicular to the wall with the trigger facing the wall. The pine board of the trap should touch the wall. Check traps each day. If you notice they've taken the bait in one area of the house but not in others, move all the traps to the area of activity. Rebait and set the traps. Dispose of any mice you catch, and repeat the whole procedure in four to five days. By waiting, you reduce the chance that a "smart mouse" will remember to avoid a trap.

- If you must use poison, use a hard plastic "bait station" that is child- and pet-resistant. Avoid boxed poison pellets. Mice can nibble the cardboard and scatter the pellets.

- Seal any opening in your home that leads from the outdoors in.

A Word on Paper

You can eliminate or substantially reduce the three main paper products in your home—paper towels, napkins, and facial tissues—by using cloth substitutes.

- Use hand and dish towels in the kitchen. Keep them separate. You don't want to dry clean dishes with a towel you mopped the counter with. (Better yet, let dishes air-dry; it's more sanitary.)

- Use cloth napkins that can be washed and reused.

- Handkerchiefs and washcloths are perfectly acceptable replacements for tissues. Even kids can use hankies in school and return them for washing. Use tissues only when someone is contagious.

- Wipe up spills with clean rags.

- When buying necessary household paper products such as toilet paper, look for a recycled brand with the highest postconsumer content possible. If you're concerned about the use of chlorine bleach in paper products, choose "totally chlorine-free" or "processed chlorine-free." (The latter refers to recycled paper only.)

This is tougher than you think. A mouse can squeeze into an opening the size of a dime. (See insulation, chapter 3.)

- Rats are bigger, smarter, and more dangerous than mice. They have been known to gnaw through the toughest substances, including concrete. If you have a rat problem, don't mess around. Hire a professional.

ONE LAST WORD . . .

As you can no doubt deduce, working with nature rather than against it is markedly safer for you and much less expensive. Give one of these remedies a try and sit back and gloat that you're no longer at the mercy of dangerous chemicals.

CHAPTER 9

GARDENING

*It is clear to me that unless we connect directly with the earth, we will not
have the faintest clue why we should save it.*
—HELEN CALDICOTT, *If You Love This Planet*

My garden is a work in progress—something I work in and something that works on me. Between the rows of tiny shoots and pepper plants, I enjoy the daily theater of bugs, weeds, sun, and
water, and I experience the direct and simple relationship between labor and reward, the practical and the spiritual. If I'm not
tending my garden, I'm certainly thinking about it. It has become
part of my life cycle, a routine destination in the circuit of my day,
a point of reference, a host of metaphors, and a wise teacher. During gardening season I'm reminded that I am a pupil of the earth.

I often visit my garden at night, with flashlight in hand or
under the glow of a full moon, looking for bugs and snails. A true
lunatic. The bugs look like tiny jewels when their eyes catch the
flashlight beam. The snails are transported by underhand flight to
another part of my backyard, and the unlucky beetles and snow-
pea-munching critters are squeezed between thumb and forefin-
ger while I mumble under my breath, "Better luck in your next
life." This drama is part of tending and guiding these edibles
toward my table. Some days there is enough to share and the
bugs, gophers, and snails enjoy the salad bar. When the plants are
young, however, life and death are determined by my watchful-
ness. It sounds hostile, brutal, and it is—especially when I need to
confront a larger garden inhabitant, like a gopher. These are a few

of the discoveries one makes when gardening: the gopher as antagonist, the snail as projectile, and ultimately the satisfaction of feeding myself and friends with the fruits of these delightful follies.

On my knees, in the dirt—eye level with the grape tendrils clinging and winding their way heavenward—I can more easily hear the voice of nature, suspend my scientific education, and experience the relatedness of all natural phenomena. To grow a tomato or a pepper and prepare a meal from your labor and care is primordially satisfying. I think the world would be radically changed if everyone had some experience with growing or raising their food. The birds sing, the peach tree blossoms, and the wind and bugs connect everything under the sun. It is at once simple and gorgeously ornate, this orchestration of life. What could be more profound than these offerings in exchange for a little care and attention?

The peach tree in my yard is the most pampered tree in the universe. All year round, I watch over it like a mother hen. Watering it in dry seasons. Spraying (organically!) when needed. And leaping into action when peach season finally arrives. I slip some air mattresses under its branches to catch the fruit when it falls. (This method is not exactly unheard-of; I know of a place where they string up tennis nets horizontally to break the fruits' fall.)

Of course I could just buy white peaches at the farmers market near home, but there's something wonderful about eating food you grew yourself. And when that crop has such a brief harvest time, it's all the more eventful. As any vegetable gardener will tell you, during the growing season you are at the mercy of the plants, and it's a delicious place to be. There are times when I think, "I know I wanted to go out to dinner tonight, but the green beans are ready!"

Some people see this as tyranny-by-chlorophyll, but I think it is quite the opposite. By choosing to grow some or all of the food you eat, you are reclaiming the power that supermarket chains and others have over what nourishes your body. You nurture the soil. You choose the seeds. You decide the price, which is hardly more than seed money, water, and a little sweat. Gardening is work, but it is also self-sufficiency.

Being able to step outside the kitchen and pick all the ingredients for a salad is a great convenience, and it means I eat better too. Gardening saves packaging. Gardening saves fuel. Organic gardening can return precious habitat for pollinating insects, birds, and other creatures. And good gardening practices reduce household food waste through composting. Beyond this, gardening can educate us and fill our lives with beauty.

For many of us the garden and farm are an abstract notion. Food is something that arrives through a small window after we've spoken into a microphone disguised as a cartoon character. The modern food industry makes it very easy to sacrifice nutrition and awareness for convenience. In this country, agriculture is dominated by agribusiness. Vertically integrated corporations control important elements of the food chain. They have established their reign over seed, fertilizer, and food systems. Trade rules, property rights, and new technologies are employed that affect genetic diversity and ultimately the safety of food. Many argue that these trends are necessary to feed the growing planet, but the more I learn about these policies, the more I realize the motives have less to do with altruism than with profit. Food *distribution*, not food *production*, is the real challenge. Efficiency, productivity, volume, price, and profit are winning out to longer-term, sustainable options that by all measures nourish not just our bodies but our souls. But it need not, as the following account shows.

THE SUBURBAN FARMER

In the dead of winter, when most of us are scouring supermarket bins in search of a tomato that doesn't taste like a tennis ball, Joan Dye Gussow is feasting on peppers she grew, picked, roasted, and froze last summer. Her Sears standing freezer, still purring after forty years, is crammed with sautéed zucchini and frozen treats such as blueberries, raspberries, and peaches. When she craves the taste of a real tomato, she reaches for a batch she sun-dried last August, or breaks out her famous roasted tomato sauce. As a rule, the majority of the fruits and veggies Gussow eats all year round come from her backyard. And no, she's not a farmer with endless acreage and a brigade of farmhands. She's a seventy-four-year-old college professor who grows enough to feed herself (and others) in a one-thousand-square-foot vegetable bed along the west bank of New York's Hudson River.

Since her college days, as she embarked on a career as a journalist, Gussow found herself increasingly interested in food, its origins, and its environmental impact. Later in life, after raising two boys, she switched gears and became a nutritionist, and she's been an eyewitness to the birth of the modern food industry. Drafted for one governmental panel after another, she's spent her career mulling over, reading, and writing about food issues.

Gussow saw reason to worry early on. Beginning in the seventies, this famously outspoken critic warned, in a string of speeches, articles, and books, that agribusiness was radically altering the way Americans eat, separating them from food tied to the season, eroding the land, destroying family farms, tainting the food supply, and consuming precious resources. "We've changed what agriculture is supposed to be," she says one summer day, taking a break from the garden. "It should be an efficient energy-capture system. Plants draw their energy from the sun and make food. Agriculture today consumes more energy than it makes, and the industry has become a dumping ground for waste. We move food around all over the place. Even someone who lives in California is not getting produce from California. They're eating food from Mexico and points south. What's the point of it? It's ridiculous, and American food is certainly not more delicious than it used to be."

In response, she began turning to the soil in her own backyard for the food she and her family ate. Always gardeners, she and her late husband, the artist Alan Gussow, began adding more and more crops to their annual repertoire. In her latest book, *This Or-*

ganic Life: Confessions of a Suburban Homesteader, she describes how she achieved what many considered impossible: to live almost entirely off the food grown in a small garden in the American Northeast. In twenty-two beds measuring three feet wide by fifteen feet long, she grows a rich assortment of veggies and herbs, not to mention berries, apples, peaches, and Asian pears. And she supplements what she grows with lamb, pork, chicken, eggs, and cured meats, all supplied by a small local farmer. She does buy rice and pasta, but never imported brands—that's how strongly she feels about eating domestically.

The food she grows on her own is carefully processed (dried, pickled, or brined) or stowed away in the freezer. She firmly believes it's easier to live this way than it was at any other time in our nation's history. "We have many methods of preservation that our parents and grandparents didn't," she says. The freezer alone allows you to stockpile food until you can get around to preserving it, thus freeing up more freezer space. (You can find terrific information and recipes for canning and preserving at www.all baking.net.)

In summer she's busy harvesting, preserving, and eating whatever the earth supplies. When autumn days become short, she tends to the garden's dwindling chores and picks the last of the fall crops. When frost kills the last of the plants, her work is done— sort of. A few hardy vegetables, such as kale or carrots, can be picked or pulled even in the dead of winter. For the most part, though, she can enjoy a three-month respite. Now, when the wind whips down the river on the way to the sea, she's nestled away indoors facing her only tough question: what do I want for dinner?

ONCE UPON A POOP

Once upon a time a cancer patient named Dom Roscioli left his job in Milwaukee and went home to his mother's Kenosha, Wisconsin, home to die. Doctors had diagnosed him with non-

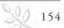

Hodgkin's lymphoma *and* a rare lung disease called sarcoidosis. Chemotherapy might have helped, but the doctors couldn't be encouraging. Dom, a Catholic diocesan priest, was only thirty-seven years old.

That was almost twenty years ago.

Father Dom, who is very much alive, now volunteers at my father's Hole in the Wall Gang camp in Ashford, Connecticut. The young campers, who suffer from leukemia and blood diseases, often beg him to tell them how he became the King of Duck Poop.

Back home in Kenosha while undergoing chemotherapy, Father Dom would hear old-timers moan about the death of their neighborhood. In the years since he'd left, Columbus Park had become home to drug dealers and gangs. Businesses closed, and addicts and dealers colonized the abandoned buildings. Night after night, sitting at his mother's kitchen, he'd hear people say, "Why don't *you* do something about it, Father?"

Father Dom thought, *What can I possibly do?* Eventually, though, he promised to try. He and his mom, along with another local pastor, pooled their money to buy a used-car lot. From that location they ran a small, nonprofit organization devoted to neighborhood improvement called Kenosha in Neighborhoods Works (KIN Works). They raised money two ways. Kids and adults brought in aluminum cans and plastic and glass bottles, which Father Dom sold directly to recycling plants. They were ahead of their time. The state of Wisconsin would not begin mandatory recycling until the mid-1990s. As the word spread, people drove in from other neighborhoods with their recyclables. They also brought along yard waste, leaves, clippings, and brush, which Father Dom sold to a waste-management company that was starting up a composting program. On the same site, he opened a small drive-in restaurant. Nothing fancy, you understand. Italian heroes. Burgers. Milk shakes. He hired people from the neighborhood to run the place and stuck his mom in the kitchen to supervise.

The money rolled in, and Father Dom's work spread to other

neighborhoods. KIN cleaned up a contaminated junkyard, shut down a porn shop near a school, and blew the whistle on a bordello run by organized crime. KIN hounded absentee landlords to fix up their properties and reported violations to the city. Father Dom's work was starting to impact the local drug trade. "It got pretty nasty for a while," he says. "We were warned off, threatened, you name it." Some officials, clearly corrupt, offered him bribes to close up shop. A thug once told him to back down or else. Father Dom, who was still in chemo, laughed at him: "What are you gonna do? You gonna have me shot? Right now, in my condition, a bullet would be a friend."

But lots of people appreciated his work. One of them, Tom Baxter, who worked at the nearby Ocean Spray cranberry-processing plant, had a proposition: "Father, can you recycle cranberry skins? I've got all you want."

Father Dom knew that food processors generate tons of food waste every year. Ocean Spray was sending it to a landfill but wanted to make a greener choice. As a sometime gardener, Father Dom knew that under the right conditions, food waste could be "cooked" into an excellent soil amendment. The only trick was finding a good source of nitrogen to accelerate decomposition. Luckily, he just happened to know a duck farmer in the next county who could help him out.

Soon mounds of duck poop and cranberry skin mash were being trucked to a twenty-acre site run by a private waste-management company. Workers mixed the two ingredients and piled it in long rows four feet high by four feet wide. There it sat for four months, while temperatures in the piles climbed to 160 degrees Fahrenheit. KIN alone had the rights to sell the finished product: rich black soil, a gardener's best friend. Father Dom employed local people, some of them disabled, to distribute the stuff, which he sold in bulk under the name Wis-Compost. Wanting to grow the business, he talked to my father, who do-

- Amount of trash thrown out by average person annually: 1,500 pounds

- Amount of trash thrown out by person who composts: 375 pounds

(Source: *Embracing the Earth*, Mark Harris)

nated the services of the team that designs all of the Newman's Own packaging.

Today the compost is sold nationwide under the name Father Dom's Duck's Doo (www.fatherdomsducksdoo.com). Sales have increased every year since its debut, helping Father Dom spread the doo—and the cash. Profits are distributed to national inner-city charities that do work similar to KIN's. Remarkably, at some point during all these adventures, Father Dom's cancer went into remission. Not sorry to see it go, he recognizes the important role it played for him in inspiring action. "The sickness became the biggest blessing of my life," he says.

Besides the restaurant, he's started a neighborhood gym, an environmental bookstore, and a gift shop called New Earth. And his charity has bought, restored, and sold ten residential and two commercial buildings.

Oddly enough, people are always calling to donate or sell him poop, which just might lead to the next big idea. Coming soon, for example, is Father Dom's Pony Express, compost made from yard waste and horse manure. In what must be an ecumenical first, Father Dom is helping a local rabbi bag and sell a chicken-manure product. And just the other day a guy called with an odd query: "Hey, Father, can you use bat guano?"

No wonder Father Dom says, "I feel like a crap magnet!"

ONCE UPON A SEED

Once upon a time, the sultan of Oman presented the Brooklyn Botanic Garden with a frankincense tree. This legendary scent, distilled from the tree's milky sap, was a luxury in ancient times, and one of the gifts of the Magi. Since trees grown in Oman produce the best perfume, the Brooklyn Botanic folks thought it would be nice to grow a few trees from cuttings and send them to other public gardens around the United States. But every snippet the gardeners tried to grow withered and died. Finally, they sent some branches to a soft-spoken New Jersey farmer named Cyrus Hyde, who coaxed them to life in no time.

Herbs and their exotic histories are Hyde's life's work. Growing up, he thought he might want to be a dairy farmer but soon learned he was allergic to cows. He tried other jobs, but nothing suited him as much as growing and drying herbs the way he'd learned from his mother. In 1966 Hyde and his wife began an herb nursery on a four-and-a-quarter-acre farm. Even in the sixties, confining a nursery to herbs was something of a gamble. But Hyde felt people who visited his own garden on the premises would instantly see the benefits of growing their own herbs. Pests seldom bother herbs, which exude a powerful scent. With a little care, a perennial plant will spring fresh from the soil each spring, and reward you with another year's worth of precious cuttings. A single plant could replace a lifetime of store-bought spices.

> *What is a weed? A plant whose virtues have not yet been discovered.*
> —*Ralph Waldo Emerson*

Hyde's gamble paid off. Thirty-six years and some land parcels later, Hyde and his family preside over Well-Sweep Herb Farm, a 120-acre nursery and mail-order business that counts among its regular customers botanical gardens in New York, Denver, and Chicago.

Hyde's zeal as a collector drives the business. While other farms might be content to offer two or three varieties of thyme, Hyde cultivates 104 varieties. It's one thing to like the taste of mint, it's another to grow 45 varieties of it. Or 75 lavenders, 62 rosemaries, and 114 types of scented geraniums.

How does he do it? Younger herbalists say that Hyde always encourages them to share their finds with other growers. Specifically, he swaps seeds and cuttings with like-minded collectors all over the country. Some would call that generosity or friendship. Hyde insists it's also good business. "We can't all grow everything," he says. "If a plant you're growing dies, at least you know where to find it." At a time when our culture and economics seem hell-bent on homogenizing plant and animal life, Hyde is keeping diversity alive. Those who visit the farm are usually stunned to find that there are so many different varieties in a single species. Apple mint. Lemon thyme. Chocolate geraniums.

Each plant, it seems, comes with a story. "This is called 'Grand Duke of Tuscany,'" Hyde will say as he twists a heavy, white blossom off a jasmine bush. "In the Middle East people stir it into chilled water for a refreshing drink." On through the brick-lined garden he goes, breaking sprigs, crushing leaves, and telling plant stories: common horsetail is such a gentle abrasive, he says, that American colonists used stalks of it to finish fine furniture. A little lovage in your potato salad, he ventures, after offering a tiny smell, and you'll never go back to celery. Spilanthes numbs tongues and gums so quickly that it was once used to treat toothaches. Syrians use zatar, which smells like oregano—"Here, sniff"—to season breads. And John the Baptist ate carob-tree pods as he wandered the desert.

President, Architect, Scientist, Organic Gardener

"I have an extensive flower border, in which I am fond of placing handsome plants or fragrant," wrote Thomas Jefferson, America's first gardener-activist. Besides his Monticello estate, the third president maintained five satellite farms, where he experimented with rarities from the Americas and abroad. He grew and ate tomatoes at a time when most Americans thought they were poisonous. He grew hemp, which he regarded as the "first necessity to the wealth and protection of the country." He dreamed of a day when American wine would rival European vintages, though his own vine experiments failed repeatedly. His famous collections are still managed today by curators at Monticello (www.monticello.org/grounds), and the on-site garden shop (www.twinleaf.org) sells heirloom seeds and live plants that Jefferson grew in his day.

At seventy-two, the milkman-turned-herbalist is still collecting and sharing seeds. To date, only one plant, possibly fictitious, eludes him. He's heard of a basil from the marshes of Lampa, Chile, whose damp leaves exude salt crystals when struck by sunlight. The omission is hardly glaring: Well-Sweep's catalog boasts forty-one basil varieties.

One day, our tour finished, Hyde spied a young friend coming up the gravel drive. "Oh, excuse me for a second," he said. "I think this fellow's come to bring me some seed."

THE DOCTOR'S GARDEN

Helen Caldicott is in the kitchen today, making a simple lunch for guests. The vegetables in her quiche come from the yard behind the house, the eggs from the chickens that busily strut about their coop. She holds off making the salad until the last second, and wanders the yard to see what's ready. One by one she picks the greens and a few sprigs of herbs.

It's autumn in Sydney, where Caldicott, who is Australian, lives. Her house is tucked onto a piece of land that was once an orange orchard, and before that a rain forest. Three years ago she bought eighty tree seedlings from a nursery and planted them in the front yard in the hope of reforesting the bush.

It was a gesture typical of a woman who has spent a lifetime caring about the earth. Regarded as the world's leading spokesperson for the antinuclear movement, Caldicott is the founder of Physicians for Social Responsibility and a nominee for the 1985 Nobel Peace Prize. The Smithsonian Institute and *Ladies' Home Journal* have both named her one of the most influential women of the twentieth century, and she's been awarded honorary degrees from nineteen universities. First and foremost, she is a doctor who has always tried to explain in simple terms what humanity's irresponsible activities could do to the fragile web of life. Her concern for our ailing planet, she has often said, is not unlike a medical person's concern for a sick patient.

"I think it's vile what they're doing to food," she says, and begins to enumerate some common practices. "They're giving the cows bovine growth hormone so they'll produce more milk, but we still don't know if that is carcinogenic. Meanwhile, the antibiotics that are routinely fed to cattle and chickens to increase their rate of growth and to prevent any infections may be contributing to the antibiotic resistance we're seeing now in human patients, and bringing about the development of resistant germs. Some of the pesticides we use are carcinogenic. Chemicals that leach from plastic bottles and others such as PCBs are ubiquitous and are estrogen mimickers. These compounds can have a feminizing effect on animals and possibly humans, and now we're see-ing birds and other animals exposed to these chemicals develop indeterminate genitalia. The fruit you buy in the store has been waxed to keep it from spoiling, so you can't really wash anything off. The chemicals are locked in. And then they're putting trout genes in strawberries. The side effects of that may take years to make themselves known."

> *No occupation is so delightful to me as the cultivation of the earth.*
> *—Thomas Jefferson*

At sixty-three, Caldicott still keeps an intense travel schedule. Flip through the TV channels someday and you may catch her debating someone on *Larry King Live*. Or patiently taking ques-tions from the audience on *Donahue*. Or reading passages from her new book, *The New Nuclear Danger,* on C-Span. And when she is through, she knows she will return to her home to sit with her grandchildren and tend her garden.

A passage she once wrote continues to inspire environmental-ists. "Hope for the earth lies not with leaders but in your own heart and soul. If you decide to save the earth, it will be saved. Each person can be as powerful as the most powerful person who ever lived—and that is you, if you love this planet."

What You Can Do

Whether you're a longtime gardener with two green thumbs or a newbie itching to try a new hobby, here are a few suggestions for earth-friendly gardening. Given the diversity of our nation's cli-mate, I can't advise you on specific plants for your neck of the woods. With the help of a good local nursery, you can decide what works best where you live. Besides, if I advised you, you'd probably end up with a forest of peach trees.

Target the chemicals first. Make a conscious effort to eliminate or minimize use of toxic pesticides, herbicides, and chemical fertilizers in your garden. Choose organic alternatives. In general, you'll feed plants with compost or composted manure and combat pests with mechanical traps, biodegradable oils, soaps, and sprays, and beneficial insects. If this is uncharted territory for you, when you visit a nursery ask for pesticides used in organic agriculture. Don't overlook obvious resources for good advice, such as the farmers you run into at organic markets or stands. Check out www.soilfoodweb.com for soil-management advice. The Web can be a wonderful resource, but as always, make every mail order count to minimize associated fuel and packaging waste. The Resources Directory lists several good sources of organic "inputs." And don't sweat it. It may be years before you can phone a mail-order company and ask with a straight face, "So, just how much guano comes in that bag?"

Banish pests on the cheap. Keep an eye out for pests as you cut flowers and pick vegetables, and use simple control methods before resorting to the big guns. (If you need help telling good bugs from bad, or if you just want to gawk at icky pictures, see the Gardens Alive and Biocontrol Network websites listed in the Resources Directory.) Gardening lore is full of homemade remedies, and in time you'll accumulate an arsenal of knowledge. For example, you can wipe aphids off plants with your hands dipped in soapy water. (Don't use antibacterial soap!) You can drown slugs by setting out small dishes of cheap beer sunk into the ground at snail's-eye level. You can sprinkle cayenne pepper around beds to keep away neighborhood pets. And you can pull up weeds as soon as you spy them, and before they scatter their seed.

Choose garden tools, supplies, and furnishings responsibly. Whether you're replacing garden items or buying them for the first time, be deliberate in your selections. Clay pots and cardboard seed trays go easy on the earth. Sturdy wood-and-steel tools last longer than flimsy plastic ones. Wood patio sets are biodegradable. Make sure, though, that you buy sustainably harvested products. (Check out Sylvania Certified, LLC, at www .certifiedwood.com for wood products that come from sustainably managed forests.) Elegant steel and cast iron are also responsible options, but you'll roast your tush sitting on 'em in Phoenix. Sturdy plastic lasts forever, but the downside is, it lasts forever. If you do buy plastic, make sure it is made of 100 percent recycled material. Go easy on the garden tchotchkes. Instead of buying "lifelike" flamingos or laughing pigs made of resin, plant flowers that attract birds, butterflies, and hummingbirds (see page 173 for suggestions).

Easy on the water. No region of the country is immune from drought and water shortages. Even if your neighborhood averages fifty inches a year, it won't all come down when you want it. And demand is forever increasing as population grows. Some simple strategies:

- Before the season starts, check hoses and water connections for leaks.

- Adjust sprinklers to water only vegetation that needs to be watered—not walkways, patios, and your napping grandma. Make sure that coverage is even.

- Help plants develop deep roots by watering deeply and infrequently. Deeper roots mean plants are healthier and better able to withstand drought. Established gardens need just one inch of water a week, so if it's rained that much, don't water. Not sure how much water you've had? Collect rain or sprinkler water in a coffee can and measure it with a ruler.

> ### Some Questions to Ask Before Buying a Plant
>
> How much sun (or shade) does it require?
>
> How tall and wide will it grow?
>
> Is it a perennial, annual, or something else?
>
> When will it bloom?
>
> Is it drought-tolerant?
>
> Is it deer-resistant?
>
> Is it invasive?

- Water in the morning or evening to avoid evaporation. Don't water on windy days.

- Consider installing a drip irrigation system. Dripping reduces evaporation and waters plants at a rate they can more easily absorb. If a drip system isn't in the cards, install a shut-off timer on your water faucet, or use a (loud) kitchen timer to tell you when to turn off the water.

- Do all you can to preserve rainwater. Place plastic rain barrels under drainspouts. Install porous paving materials—brick, granite, or gravel—on walkways to absorb rather than repel rainwater. If your property is sloped, use terraces and retaining walls.

- Use mulch and compost to improve your soil's water-holding capacity. (I'll discuss both in greater detail later.) Briefly, mulch is a thick layer of organic matter—wood chips, dried nutshells, shredded bark—spread on plant beds to shield the soil from the sun and retain moisture. Compost is well-rotted vegetation—from grass clippings and dead leaves to last summer's leftover salad—that is added to soil to improve fertility.

- During drought emergencies, water plants from most precious to least. In any landscape, older, bigger plantings cost more to replace. Dead trees and large shrubs can even cost a bundle to remove. If push comes to shove, water in this order: trees, shrubs, perennials, annuals, containers, and lawn.

Rethink the lawn. We Americans lavish more than thirty billion dollars a year on our precious plots of green. Thirty percent of all water consumed on the East Coast, and 60 percent on the West, goes to lawns. Seventy million pounds of chemicals are dumped on lawns each year to kill weeds or pests, much of it washing into our water supply when it rains. The mowers we use to tame this bland wilderness emit as much hydrocarbon in an hour as a car driven fifty miles. And tons of clippings end up in a landfill when they could easily feed our soil. Believe me, I enjoy lawns; as a playing and walking surface, grass can't be beat. But for our own health, we must start treating lawns as extensions of our organic houses and gardens. Besides fertilizing and treating weeds organically, you can make a difference by doing the following:

- Raise your mower blades to the highest setting. Ideally, you want to cut only the top third of the grass. Let the clippings fall and be recycled into the lawn. Tall grass shades out weeds and develops stronger roots. Taller grass also grows more slowly between cuttings because it isn't rushing to produce more food by photosynthesis. This method requires you to mow more frequently, lest you're left with heaps of clippings that smother the lawn.

- Some lawn mowers will mulch the grass clippings. If not, utilitize what you have in your compost pile or as a very thin layer (less than one inch) on any bare surface in your garden. Clippings added to compost piles must be mixed with dry organic matter to reduce odors and matting.

- Cut back on water usage. At the height of summer, your grass will naturally brown. But don't worry. It's remarkably resilient and will return. Really.

- If you hate lawn care, maybe you're ready to start reducing the size of your lawn. You could replace part of it with flowers and shrubs, or even a low-maintenance ground cover. If you need a play area for children and pets, you could replace a swath of lawn with soft, shredded bark.

- If you do reduce your lawn, you can then switch to a nonmotorized reel mower and never buy gasoline again. One caveat: not all reel mowers cut tall grass well. Check the height range before buying.

Go native, and xeriscape: Wherever you live, it's better to plant species native to your area. In particular, look for drought-tolerant plants. Choosing plants that thrive on little or no supplemental moisture is called xeriscaping. When you design your garden, group together plants with similar watering needs so you can water the whole bed as necessary instead of singling out individual plants. Obviously, drought-tolerant varieties should go in the driest, sunniest spots in your garden. If the plants are new, water them regularly for the first six months to a year until they are established. Then you can reduce watering.

Just starting out? Avoid spending a lot of money until you know your property well. Take time to locate the sunny and shady spots. Look for places that get about six to eight hours of sun a day. Those are the best spots for vegetable patches and herb gardens. At first you might want to stick to vegetables such as tomatoes and peppers, herbs such as basil, and easy flowering annuals such as marigolds, petunias, impatiens, and geraniums. Sunflowers are fun to start from seed. Don't be afraid to plant similar plants in different spots, just to see how well they do. Next year you'll build on what you've learned about your property. Some other pointers:

- Know your zone. North America is divided into eleven different growing regions, or hardiness zones. A plant rated "to zone 5" will survive winters down to −15 degrees Fahrenheit. It's essential to know your zone when choosing perennials, shrubs, and trees. To find out what zone you're in, see the National Arboretum's website (www.usna.usda.gov/Hardzone/ushzmap .html).

- Within each zone, state land-grant universities dispense local gardening and agricultural information free of charge. You can

Drought-Tolerant Plants

I list a few here only to show that such a strategy is not limiting. Remember that plants ideal for xeriscaping in Kennebunkport, Maine, would be darn thirsty in Moab, Utah. Only a good local nursery can guide your selections.

Shrubs and Trees

Bayberry

Bluebeard (*Caryopteris*)

Broom

Butterfly bush (*Buddleia*)

Crab apple

Crimson pygmy barberry

Hawthorn

Holly (*Ilex*)

Juniper

Linden

Maple (hedge, *Amur*)

Mock orange

Norway spruce

Privet

Rose of Sharon

Viburnum

Winterberry

Yucca

Perennials

Acanthus

Artemisia

Aster

Bee balm (*Monarda*)

Bellflower (*Campanula*)

Black-eyed Susan (*Rudbeckia*)

Blanketflower (*Gaillardia*

Butterfly weed (*Asclepias*)

Chamomile

Coneflower (*Echinacea*)

Coreopsis

Daisies (*Anthemis, Chrysanthemum, Leucanthemum*)

Delphinium

Geranium

Grasses

Jerusalem artichoke

Lady's mantle (*Alchemilla*)

Lamb's ears (*Stachys*)

Lavender

Lupine

Mallow (*Malva*)

Marjoram

Mullein (*Verbascum*))

Oregano

Penstemon

Phlox (creeping)

Rue

Russian sage (*Perovskia*)

Sage (culinary)

Sedum

St.-John's-wort (*Hypericum*)

Yarrow (*Achillea*)

Terms to Know

Annuals: These plants complete their life cycle in a single growing season. Flowering annuals, for example, blossom continuously until the plant experiences a killing frost. Vegetables are annuals.

Perennials: These plants live at least three years. They go dormant in winter and return in spring. A flowering perennial may only blossom during a brief period of time, so gardeners must rely on other plants to provide color during the off months. Many herbs are perennials.

Biennials: This plant produces leaves the first year and flowers the second. It usually re-seeds itself about the time it dies.

Hardy annuals: These plants live one season, blossom continuously, and reseed themselves for next year.

Tender perennials: These perennials cannot take frost or freezing. They are plants living outside their zone, and they rely on doting owners to shelter them indoors during winter. (Think of a potted citrus tree in Michigan.) Unless you're willing to do this, try to avoid collecting (too many) exotics.

find your local cooperative extension office at CRSEES (www.reeusda.gov/1700/statepartners/usa.htm).

- Before you go on a plant-buying spree, think about how you might use your garden. Do you cook a lot? An herb garden containing two or three herbs you use often might be just the thing. Do you have kids and pets? You might focus on designing a more appropriate place for them to run around. Do you just want to make sure your dirt doesn't blow away? Ask a nursery specialist to direct you to low-maintenance plants and ground covers, or the nearest gravel heap.

- While you're mulling over your future Eden, take time to improve the soil. Soil types vary from region to region, tending to extremes of too much sand or clay. To start out on the right foot, you might get your soil tested to see what it really needs.

The ideal is black, friable soil. To get it that way, you'll need to add organic matter such as leaf mold (wet, rotting leaves), well-rotted manure, or compost. Even if you don't intend to plant until next season, start adding the good stuff now. You might experiment with a nourishing cover crop.

- If you have little or no earth to call your own, you can easily plant a beautiful container garden. Keep in mind, though, that potted plants require more frequent watering, since plant roots are unable to grow ever deeper in search of moisture.

- Looking for design ideas? Instead of emptying your wallet on gardening books and magazines, make time to visit local public gardens. Then, for contrast, plan a hike or visit to a nature preserve. In these two settings alone, you'll see the difference between gardens designed by humans and gardens designed by nature. The challenge—and part of the fun—is incorporating lessons from both.

- Not enough space or time to garden? Find a community garden and donate your time or money.

Learn to make compost. Mulch, mulch, mulch! If you take a walk in the woods, you'll notice a wealth of crumbly black soil. As leaves and dead plants pile up, they are broken down by worms and microorganisms, which feast on the endless buffet and turn it into dirt. This simple feat, nature's recycling method, is the cornerstone of organic gardening. Nothing humans can cook up in a lab is as nutritious for growing plants as this soil, or humus ("hyoo-mus"). Organic farmers and gardeners mimic this process. They save dead plants generated on their property and compost them to make humus. They mix the stuff directly into their fields or garden beds. Sometimes they lay it in a thick "mulch" layer over the earth.

Compost improves soil structure, texture, and aeration and helps soil retain moisture; it feeds plants the way they are designed by nature to be fed; it adds microscopic critters to the soil that break down dead matter into easily accessible nutrients. When properly made, compost is disease-, pest-, and weed-free.

Mulch is a thick "blanket" that covers the top of the soil; it can be made from wood chips, grass clippings, hay, leaves, shells, pebbles, or even sheets of plastic; it absorbs water and keeps it from eroding soil; it shields sensitive roots from the heat of the sun; and it blocks weeds from popping up. Compost is the best mulch around.

By now you're thinking, "How can I get me some compost?" The cheapest, most reliable way is to make it yourself.

Whether you know it or not, you're sitting on a wealth of it. About one third of all household trash is organic waste. Carrot tops and peelings. Banana skins. Apple cores. Wilted lettuce leaves. Eggshells. Tea bags. Coffee grounds. Garlic skins. Grass clippings. Dead (but not diseased) leaves and plants. All of this stuff, which we Americans are accustomed to sending to a landfill, can be turned into free fertilizer for our gardens.

You need a place in your yard to set up a compost bin. Before you buy or make one, check with your town. Many cities now offer bins free to residents, in an effort to reduce landfill waste. The most common setup is a three-sided wooden stall. Other folks set up two stalls side by side and happily hurl stuff back and forth between the two with a pitchfork like a bartender mixing drinks. You don't even have to build your own these days. Companies such as Real Goods (www.realgoods.com), Gardener's Supply (www.gardeners.com), and a host of others sell upright and tumbling composters made of tough plastic. I use a tumbler. I toss in my kitchen and yard scraps and roll the thing around my yard. I probably look goofy doing it, but it works. Spinners and tumblers are excellent options if you have close neighbors or are concerned about attracting critters; because they are sealed, animals can't get in to scavenge.

Compost calls for four ingredients: oxygen, water, carbon, and nitrogen. The first two are easy; the second two always confuse people. Simply put, carbon is any dry, brown material such as leaves, straw, brown paper bags, or strips of newspaper. Nitrogen, on the other hand, is the green, protein-rich material such as freshly plucked weeds and plants, grass clippings, household fruits and veggies. The manure of chickens, cows, and sheep is also rich in nitrogen. (I know: they're not green, but they sure are ripe!)

A Child's Garden

Planting and tending a garden with young children can be a truly magical experience. Your backyard becomes an all-in-one classroom, zoo, and snack bar. Kids will happily help out, provided they don't have to wait all season for rewards. To keep them interested, plant quick-growing veggies, fruit-bearing shrubs, and large, flashy flowers that will delight kids and attract wildlife. When starting plants from seed, choose varieties whose seeds are easily handled by small fingers.

Fruit: Ever-bearing or alpine strawberries are easy. Seasoned gardeners may want to tackle blueberries and raspberries.

Herbs: Basil, parsley, and scented geraniums.

Flowering plants: Butterfly bush, butterfly weed, morning glories, black-eyed Susans, and edible varieties such as honeysuckle and sunflowers.

Veggies: Cherry tomatoes, pickling cucumbers, pole beans, leaf lettuce, peas, carrots, beets, onions (from sets), and radishes.

Structures: Window boxes, hummingbird and bird feeders, birdhouses, birdbaths, or fountains.

To build a pile in a bin, you alternate layers of browns and greens, sprinkle on a little water to moisten the pile, and cover the whole enchilada with a tarp when you reach the top. If you have a tumbler, you toss scraps in willy-nilly, moisten it, and roll it around. In both cases, microbes begin feasting on the goop, and as they burn the calories, the temperature of the pile heats up.

Remember how Father Dom's compost "cooked" at 160 degrees? Well, compost piles can really get that hot on summer days. The higher the temperature, the faster decomposition goes. At higher temperatures, pests and weed seeds die, but the microbes live on. In fact, when the pile cools off to 90 or 100 degrees

Fahrenheit (they actually sell huge thermometers that allow you to test it), it means those little bad boys are kicking back from the dinner table, begging for more. By then the pile will have shrunk, and you need to turn it to serve up what they've missed. Eventually, you'll get to the point where the temperature won't budge, regardless of how much you turn it. That's when it's done.

For composting to work, the pile's carbon-nitrogen ratio should be twenty to one. To make this more complicated, not all browns and greens are created equal. For example, dry leaves and sawdust are both considered browns, but sawdust contains eight times more carbon. If you mix the batches in different ratios (and we all do), the composting process stalls. Don't be discouraged if you can't get your pile to heat up properly. I've had a tough time turning my scraps into "black gold." More often, I get dirt with chunks of undigested produce and need to adjust the mix. Stick with it. A little common sense usually sets the pile to rights. It might help to remember this little poem:

Too much brown, composting slows down.
Too much green, the pile smells like a latrine.

What can you do if it's just not working?

- The rate of decomposition varies among ingredients. A moldy carrot takes longer to break down than a lettuce leaf. Help things move along by chopping kitchen scraps well before tossing them on the pile.

- Consider building a bigger pile. An optimal pile is three feet square.

- The material should feel only as damp as a wrung sponge. If it's too dry, wet it. When done properly, compost piles don't smell.

If yours is malodorous, it's probably too wet. Aerate and add some more dry brown material.

What about composting in winter? It depends how much you want to work. Composting stops in cold weather, but determined gardeners feed their scraps indoors to worms, or insulate their outdoor bins with straw to lock in heat, or compost in the garage in trash pails. (Worm bins are also a good choice for apartment dwellers.) For more suggestions, see the Compost Resource Page website (www.oldgrowth.org/compost).

Encourage wildlife. An organic garden can provide a much-needed oasis for beneficial insects, butterflies, bees, and birds, not to mention the occasional insect-gobbling toad or turtle. Anything larger and you risk subsidizing the meal plans of countless woodland creatures. Take the necessary precautions. Fence out deer and burrowing creatures. Keep a fine net handy to throw over fruit-bearing shrubs when they ripen. (Birds always seem to know the exact day!) Do encourage visits from pollinating insects by planting flowers in and around your vegetable garden. These creatures are essential to the productivity of your crops. Bees, birds, and butterflies all need water. A birdbath or shallow pool will be appreciated by your guests. Just remember to clean it weekly and refresh the water frequently to avoid breeding mosquitoes.

Bees enjoy asters, bee balm, cosmos, geranium, lavender, mint, poppies, rosemary, sage, sunflowers, thyme, and zinnias.

Butterflies enjoy alyssum, butterfly bush, calendula, daylilies, fennel, hollyhocks, marigolds, phlox, and shasta daisies. (Butterflies also lay eggs, in which case you'll find their caterpillar offspring munching on your plants. An extra bed of parsley is more than enough to sate their appetites. Or consider planting borage, fennel, milkweed, nettle, or thistle.)

Hummingbirds enjoy ajuga, butterfly weed, columbine, bleeding heart, foxgloves, lobelia, poppies, phlox, and veronica.

Become a seed saver. Thrifty gardeners save seeds each season so they don't have to buy new ones in the coming year. Besides this obvious benefit, seed saving is a time-honored way of preserving plant diversity. At a time when small seed companies are being gobbled up by large corporations intent on patenting genetic material, you can help out by doing three things: save your seed, swap seed with other gardeners, and patronize small, independent

An Eclectic Mix

Scott Chaskey, whom you met in chapter 1, is an organic farmer, home gardener, and poet. His picks for favorite plants include the following.

Beets: "They're really extraordinary in autumn when the weather cools and they get sweet. And you can eat the tops too!"

Borage: "I love this herb. It's an edible flower that you can use in salad. It tastes like cucumber."

Buckwheat: "I plant it as a cover crop. Seeing it out in the field, three feet high, white flowers, covered with insects, is pretty much what a plant is for me."

Cosmos (annual flower): "I know they're simple and gaudy, but I like them. Last year I planted a long hedge of them, and people would immerse themselves in these six-foot plants and come out happy."

Garlic: "It's really easy to grow. You just break off cloves and plant them in the fall, and harvest them next summer when only five leaves are green."

Potatoes: "Grow fingerlings. They're good and prolific, and it feels good to get your food that way, digging in the soil for them."

seed companies. Each year try a few heirloom varieties just for fun, and pass those seeds along. Wherever possible, choose seeds that are organic and untreated (not sprayed with fungicides). Some plants grow more easily from cuttings, so be open to that avenue as well. Never take cuttings or entire plants from public lands and wilderness areas.

See the Resources Directory for seed-swapping and seed-company listings.

Scavenge wildly and proudly. Serious gardeners are as opportunistic as garden pests. If they spy a wooden clothes dryer in a neighbor's trash, they'll fish it out. Instant garden stakes! The same green thumb that cultivates roses can transform a plastic soda bottle into a bird feeder or an irrigation tool. Don't ever be ashamed of repurposing your honest finds this way. This is reducing, reusing, and recycling at its best. Now, which of you borrowed my bypass pruners?

One Last Word . . .

I like what Joan Gussow says about agriculture being an "energy-capture" system. Plants have evolved the most efficient energy system ever devised. They convert photons, particles of light, into food. When they die, they scatter their seed and fertilize a new generation. Nothing is wasted. Everything is recycled. If left alone, this cycle will repeat itself forever.

If you plant a garden, you cannot help but absorb that lesson. You're schooled in it every day, as you watch flowers bloom, pick your vegetables, and stack the compost pile ever higher. When you leave the garden, you take the lessons with you. Organic gardening is like that; it guides you in ways you cannot predict. You shun chemicals because you don't want them around your water and soil. If it doesn't rain, you'll feel compelled to conserve water. You'll take an interest in renewable energy too, because it all feels connected somehow. And it is.

EPILOGUE: GENEROSITY

You must be the change you wish to see in the world.
—Mahatma Gandhi

Whatever you can do or dream, begin it.
Boldness has genius, power and magic in it.
—Goethe

My mother and father are both very accomplished people. But they didn't always appear that way to me. For most of my life they were just Ma and Pa. The change in perspective occurred when, as an adult, I determined that I wanted to make a difference, however small, and give something back. I realized I had a gift, but the gift wasn't the privilege of being born to creative parents who supplied me with opportunities, security, and care. The gift grew out of watching my parents—their actions and the choices they've made throughout their lives. What I saw was humility and generosity.

If you were to ask my father about his remarkable success with acting, racing cars, and starting a food company, he would simply reply, "Luck." I think, though, that luck is the by-product of determination and a heap of hard work. My mother too, working her magic onstage, is unassuming about her achievements—not the least of which was raising a family.

My parents' humility shapes their generosity toward others. They believe that with good fortune comes responsibility. This isn't a family mantra, or the stated motivation behind my father's choice, and mine, to give all profits from Newman's Own

Organics to charity. What my parents discovered, and teach me still, is that the secret to a good life is giving. In a way, we give for selfish reasons: it's fulfilling and meaningful, and it brings us joy.

"All profits to charity" wasn't an idea my father stumbled on one day as a marketing concept. Not until the company's second year would he even allow that fact to be printed on the product labels, and then only in small type. To my pa, proclaiming his generosity was somehow unnecessary and cheapened the concept. "True generosity," he would say, "is done anonymously." In the end, he was persuaded that letting other people know where the profits are going allows them to participate.

My father would also say that the highest form of generosity is to give someone a job and purposeful work. Certainly transforming a salad-dressing recipe into a food company with estimated sales in 2002 of $125 million has provided a few jobs along the way, from farmers and truckers to packers and distributors. Many families are involved in the Newman's Own enterprise, and charity dollars have reached many of their communities.

But generosity encompasses more than giving. It's a way of living. It's a particular attitude toward oneself, other people, animals, plants, and all things. Generosity is the act of honoring, respecting, and appreciating what you and others have. It is refusing to detract from or diminish someone else's hope or joy. Acknowledging another person's good fortune with a smile is an act of generosity. Spending an hour with someone in need is generosity. Choosing not to ignore the suffering of others is generosity. Generosity in this sense is the opposite of exploitation.

Attempting to live according to high ideals is inevitably somewhat frustrating and sometimes disappointing. As Pete Seeger said at eighty-two, "I've come to the conclusion that there is nothing good that doesn't have bad consequences and nothing bad that doesn't have good consequences." Humility was my first corporate lesson—accepting the realities and limitations of a business built on ecological and alternative principles but necessarily operating under conventional constraints. We use energy, transportation, and packaging to sell our products while doing our best to make choices that minimize the impact of these necessities. Still, at Newman's Own Organics we must be open to constant evaluation. Self-criticism must be policy and a form of corporate humility. We are not free of all wrongdoing because we support organic farming and give our profits to charity. In fact, we are even more accountable because of our goals.

My friend and the founder of Patagonia, Inc., Yvon Chouinard, expressed the dilemma another way when he proclaimed about his environmentally responsible clothing company, "Everything we make pollutes." After examination he realized the best antidote for that admission was quality. "The most responsible thing we can do is to make each product as well as we know how so it lasts as long as possible." Tossing in the corporate towel, giving up his company to pursue a life of surfing, however attractive to Yvon (and to me, for that matter), would quickly become massively unsatisfying.

Most of us associate generosity with money. Financial donations certainly are one expression of generosity. Patagonia gives 1 percent of sales, or 10 percent of pretax profit, whichever is greater, to environmental causes. Since 1985 they have given more than $17 million. In the twenty years since its founding, Newman's Own has given $200 million to educational and environmental charities. But these companies and many others that are similarly structured have an impact not only because of their dollar contributions to worthy causes but because they influence other businesses, consumers, and policies for the good.

And did I mention that I like what I do because it's personally rewarding? In this context I meet and befriend some of the most interesting, bighearted, vibrant people around. My relationships with farmers, colleagues, natural-food-store owners, and chefs, among others, give my work meaning. The more I try to encourage others, the more inspired I am. Giving *of* yourself is also a way to give *to* yourself. Whether you are a student, a homemaker, a plumber, or a banker, you can nurture those around you. No doubt you've noticed this already: the distinctions between you and me, us and them, mine and yours dissolve when you share.

I realize what a small impact we have made at Newman's Own Organics, and how far we need to go, but it's better than nothing. Something, anything, you do is better than nothing. The value of whatever action you take is measured not just in terms of impact but also by the integrity of your intent.

These are big ideas—starting companies, charitable giving, organic farming, helping communities—but big ideas begin small. They often start with an individual with a generous spirit, something we can all cultivate. The only requirement is the will to do so. It's something one can practice and get good at.

Cultivating a generous spirit starts with mindfulness. Mindfulness, simply stated, means paying attention to what is actually happening; it's about what is really going on. It's being aware of what you are doing and experiencing, and how that affects others. You can call it karma, or reaping what you sow, or something that is summed up by the expression "what goes around comes around." The point is, what you put out not only affects the world around you, it affects the way you are in the world.

On the other hand, if you are not aware of your intentions or the results of your actions, you can easily lose your moorings, drifting along until, one day, you can't figure out where you are or how you got there. Or you might achieve your goals but miss out on the process, which is what makes up most of life. A person with a generous spirit appreciates the moment and offers thanks somehow, creatively, any way that comes to mind—listening to a friend, letting another driver in, making eye contact with the person at the cash register, teaching someone how to read.

Many of the issues we discuss in this book are large and complicated. But a good life is not strictly defined by one's contribution toward solving the giant problems, nor is chaining yourself to a tree required. You can start where you are: speak the truth, respect others, take responsibility for yourself. The good that radiates will affect you, then your neighbor, then your community, your government, and the world. A generous spirit is contagious.

My pa once said, "If people knew how good it feels to give something away, they wouldn't wait until they die to do it." At the end of the day, it's probably not what you amassed but what you gave away that will bring you joy. Generosity is not the fruit of a good life; it is the only path to achieving one.

Resources Directory

CHAPTER 1: FOOD

Restaurants

Chez Panisse
1517 Shattuck Avenue
Berkeley, CA 94709
Café reservations: (510) 548-5049
Restaurant reservations:
   (510) 548-5525
Website: www.chezpanisse.com

Frontera Grill
Topolobampo
445 North Clark Street
Chicago, IL 60610
Tel.: (312) 661-1434
Fax: (312) 661-1830
Website: www.fronterakitchens.com

Advocacy Groups and Agencies

USDA's National Organic Program
Richard Mathews, Program Manager
USDA-AMS-TMP-NOP

Room 4008–South Building
1400 and Independence Avenue SW
Washington, DC 20250-0020
Tel.: (202) 720-3252
Fax: (202) 205-7808
E-mail: NOPWebmaster@usda.gov
Website: www.ams.usda.gov/nop/
   index.htm

Oregon Tilth
470 Lancaster Drive NE
Salem, OR 97301
Tel.: (503) 378-0690
Fax: (503) 378-0809
Website: www.tilth.org

Worldwatch Institute
1776 Massachusetts Avenue NW
Washington, DC 20036-1904
Tel.: (202) 452-1999
Fax: (202) 296-7365
E-mail: worldwatch@worldwatch.org
Website: www.worldwatch.org

Environmental Working Group
1718 Connecticut Avenue NW,
    Suite 600
Washington, DC 20009
Tel.: (202) 667-6982
Fax: (202) 232-2592
E-mail: info@ewg.org
Website: www.ewg.org

Chef's Collaborative
441 Stuart Street, #712
Boston, MA 02116
Tel.: (617) 236-5200
E-mail: cc2000@chefnet.com
Website: www.chefnet.com/cc2000

Share Our Strength
733 Fifteenth Street NW, Suite 640
Washington, DC 20005
Tel.: (800) 969-4767
Fax: (202) 347-5868
Website: www.strength.org

Organic Farming Research
    Foundation
P.O. Box 440
Santa Cruz, CA 95061
Tel.: (831) 426-6606
Fax: (831) 426-6670
E-mail: research@ofrf.org
Website: www.ofrf.org

Natural-Food Stores

Wild Oats Community Markets, Inc.
3375 Mitchell Lane
Boulder, CO 80301
Tel.: (303) 440-5220
Fax: (303) 928-0022;
    (800) 494-WILD (9453)

E-mail: info@wildoats.com
Website: www.wildoats.com

Whole Foods Market
601 North Lamar, Suite 300
Austin, TX 78703
Tel.: (512) 477-4455
E-mail: rs.team@wholefoods.com
Website: www.wholefoods.com

Organic Meat and Poultry

Eat Wild
State-by-state database of organic meat
    and poultry farmers
Website: www.eatwild.com

Slanker's Grass-Fed Meats
R.R. 2, Box 175
Powderly, TX 75473
Tel.: (903) 732-4653 (office); toll-free:
    (866) SLANKER (752-6537)
E-mail: goodmeat@slanker.com
Website: www.texasgrassfedbeef.com

Community Supported Agriculture

Local Harvest
State-by-state database of CSAs
E-mail: partners@localharvest.org
Website: www.localharvest.org

Robyn Van En Center for CSA
    Resources
Wilson College
Fulton Center for Sustainable Living
1015 Philadelphia Avenue
Chambersburg, PA 17201
Contact: Stephanie Reph
Tel.: (717) 264-4141 ext. 3352

Fax: (717) 264-1578
E-mail: info@csacenter.org
Website: www.csacenter.org

Quail Hill Farm
Peconic Land Trust
296 Hampton Road
P.O. Box 1776
Southampton, NY 11969
Tel.: (631) 283-3195
Fax: (631) 283-0235
E-mail: PLT@PeconicLandTrust.org
Website: www.peconiclandtrust.org

Organic Food by Mail

Diamond Organics
P.O. Box 2159
Freedom, CA 95019
Tel.: (888) ORGANIC (674-2642)
Fax: (888) 888-6777
E-mail: info@diamondorganics.com
Website: www.diamondorganics.com

Organic Wholesalers/Buying-Club Options

Federation of Ohio River Cooperatives
320-E Outerbelt Street
Columbus, OH 43213-1597
Tel.: (614) 861-2446; toll-free:
    (888) WE-OWN-IT (936-9648)
Fax: (614) 861-7638
E-mail: customerservice@
    forcwarehouse.com
Website: www.forcwarehouse.com

Mountain Peoples Warehouse
New accounts: toll-free:
    (800) 679-8735

Tel.: (530) 889-9544
Fax: (530) 889-9544
Website: www.mtnpeopleswhs.com

Blooming Prairie
Blooming Prairie Warehouse
2340 Heinz Road
Iowa City, IA 52240
Tel.: (319) 337-6448

Blooming Prairie Natural Foods
510 Kasota Avenue SE
Minneapolis, MN 55414
Tel.: (612) 378-9774
Website: www.bpco-op.com

Ozark Cooperative
P.O. Box 1528
Fayetteville, AR 72702
Tel.: (479) 521-4920
Fax: (479) 521-9100
E-mail: warehouse@ozark.coop
Website: www.ozarkcoop.com

North Farm Cooperative
204 Regas Road
Madison, WI 53714
Tel.: (608) 241-2667; toll-free:
    (800) 236-5880
Fax: (608) 241-0688
E-mail: nfcoop@northfarm.com
Website: www.northfarm.com

Northeast Cooperatives
90 Technology Drive
P.O. Box 8188
Brattleboro, VT 05304-8188
Tel.: (802) 257-5856; toll-free:
    (800) 334-9939
Website: www.northeastcoop.com

Neshaminy Valley Natural Food
5 Louise Drive
Ivyland, PA 18974
Tel.: (215) 443-5545; toll-free:
    (800) 950-1009

Food Coop
Online resource for coop information
    and listings
Website: www.foodcoop.net

Coop Directory Service
1254 Etna Street
St. Paul, MN 55106
Tel. and Fax: (651) 774-9189
E-mail: thegang@coopdirectory.org
Website: www.coopdirectory.org

Fair-Trade Coffee/Chocolate

Global Exchange
2017 Mission Street #303
San Francisco, CA 94110
Tel.: (415) 255-7296
Fax: (415) 255-7498
E-mail: info@globalexchange.org
Website: www.globalexchange.org

Organic Wine and Beer

Organic Vintners
1911 Eleventh Street, Suite 203
Boulder, CO 80302
Tel.: toll-free (800) 216-3898
Fax: (303) 245-8911
E-mail: info@organicvintners.com
Website: www.organicvintners.com

Organic Wine Press
175 Second Street
Bandon, OR 97411
Tel.: (541) 347-3326
Website: www.organicwinepress.com

Wolaver's Organic Beer
793 Exchange Street
Middlebury, VT 05753
Tel.: toll-free (800) 473-0727
E-mail: info@wolavers.com
Website: www.wolavers.com

Pacific Western Brewing Co.
641 North Nechako Road
Prince George, BC
Canada V2K 4M4
Tel.: (250) 562-2424
Fax: (250) 562-0799
E-mail: mail@pwbrewing.com
Website: www.pwbrewing.com

Frederick Brewing Co.
4607 Wedgewood Boulevard
Frederick, MD 21703
Tel.: (301) 694-7899
Website: www.fredbrew.com

New Belgium Brewing
500 Linden Street
Fort Collins, CO 80524
Tel.: (970) 221-0524; toll-free:
    (888) NBB-4044
Fax: (970) 221-0535
E-mail: nbb@newbelgium.com
Website: www.newbelgium.com

CHAPTER 2: TRANSPORTATION

Auto Companies

General Motors Electric Car
Tel.: toll-free (800) 25-ELECTRIC
Website: www.gmev.com

Ford Motor Company
Customer Relationship Center
P.O. Box 6248
Dearborn, MI 48126
Tel.: toll-free (800) 392-3673

Think Mobility Electric Vehicles
Website: www.thinkmobility.com

Ford Escape Hybrid Electric Vehicle
Website: www.hybridford.com

American Honda Motor Co.
Honda Automobile Customer Service
1919 Torrance Boulevard
Mail Stop: 500-2N-7D
Torrance, CA 90501-2746
Tel.: toll-free (800) 999-1009
Fax: (310) 783-3023 (24 hours)
General website: www.hondacars.com
Civic Hybrid:
    www.civichybrid.honda.com
Honda Insight:
    www.hondacars.com/models/
    insight

Toyota
1919 Torrance Boulevard
Torrance, CA 90501-2746
Tel.: toll-free (800) GO TOYOTA
General website: www.toyota.com

Toyota Prius:
    www.toyota.com/html/shop/
    vehicles/prius
Rav4 Electric Vehicle:
    www.rav4ev.toyota.com

Electric Cars

Electric Vehicle Association of
    America
701 Pennsylvania Avenue NW
Third Floor, East Building
Washington, DC 20004
Tel.: (202) 508-5995
Fax: (202) 508-5924
Website: www.evaa.org

Consumer Guide

Green Book: Environmental Guide to
    Cars and Trucks
American Council for an Energy-
    Efficient Economy
1001 Connecticut Avenue NW,
    Suite 801
Washington, DC 20036
Tel.: (202) 429-8873
Fax: (202) 429-2248
E-mail: info@aceee.org
Website: www.greenercars.com

Designers

Hypercar, Inc.
110 Midland Avenue, Suite 202
Basalt, CO 81621
Tel.: (970) 927-4556
E-mail: info@hypercar.com
Website: www.hypercar.com

Green Auto Rental

Environmental Rental Car Company
Tel.: (877) EV-RENTAL
Website: www.evrental.com

CHAPTER 3: ENERGY AND WATER

Foam Recycling

Alliance of Foam Packaging Recyclers
1298 Cronson Boulevard, Suite 201
Crofton, MD 21114
Tel.: (410) 451-8340
Fax: (410) 451-8343
Website: www.epspackaging.org

Advocacy Groups and Agencies

American Council for an Energy-
  Efficient Economy
1001 Connecticut Avenue NW,
  Suite 801
Washington, DC 20036
Tel.: (202) 429-8873
Fax: (202) 429-2248
E-mail: info@aceee.org
Website: www.aceee.org

Energy Star
Tel.: (888) STAR YES (782-7937)
Website: www.energystar.gov

Green-e
Center for Resource Solutions
Presidio Building
49 Moraga Avenue
P.O. Box 29512
San Francisco, CA 94129
Tel.: (888) 634-7336
Fax: (415) 561-2105
Website: www.green-e.org

Department of Energy's Green Power
  Network
Website: www.eren.doe.gov/
  greenpower

Real Goods Solar Living Center
13771 South Highway 101
P.O. Box 836
Hopland, CA 95449
Website: www.solarliving.org

Building Supplies

North American Insulation Manufac-
  turers Association
44 Canal Center Plaza, Suite 310
Alexandria, VA 22314
Tel.: (703) 684-0084
Fax: (703) 684-0427
E-mail: insulation@naima.org
Website: www.simplyinsulate.com

Efficient Windows Collaborative Pro-
  gram Manager
Alliance to Save Energy
1200 Eighteenth Street NW, Suite 900
Washington, DC 20036
Tel.: (202) 530-2245
Fax: (202) 331-9588
Website: www.efficientwindows.org

National Fenestration Rating Council
8484 Georgia Avenue, Suite 320

Silver Spring, MD 20910
Tel.: (301) 589-1776
Fax: (301) 589-3884
E-mail: info@nfrc.org
Website: www.nfrc.org

Refrigerators

Sunfrost
P.O. Box 1101
Arcata, CA 95518
Tel.: (707) 822-9095
Fax: (707) 822-6213; (707) 822-9095
E-mail: info@sunfrost.com
Website: www.sunfrost.com

Compact-Fluorescent Lightbulbs

Philips Lighting Co.
200 Franklin Square Drive
Somerset, NJ 08875-6800
Tel.: toll-free (800) 555-0050
Website:
    www.lighting.philips.com/nam/
    feature/marathon

Retailer

Gaiam Real Goods
360 Interlocken Boulevard, Suite 300
Broomfield, CO 80021-3440
Tel.: toll-free (800) 762-7325
Website: www.realgoods.com

Water-Purification Manufacturers

Culligan International
1 Culligan Parkway
Northbrook, IL 60062-6209
Tel.: (847) 205-6000

E-mail: feedback@culligan.com
Website: www.culligan.com

BRITA Products Company
P.O. Box 24305
Oakland, CA 94623-9981
Tel.: toll-free (800) 24-BRITA
Website: www.brita.com

PUR
9300 North Seventy-fifth Avenue
Minneapolis, MN 55428
Tel.: toll-free (800) PUR-LINE
    (787-5463)
Website: www.purwater.com

Water-Purification Certification

NSF International
P.O. Box 130140
789 North Dixboro Road
Ann Arbor, MI 48113-0140
Tel.: (734) 769-8010; toll-free:
    (800) NSF-MARK
Fax: (734) 769-0109
E-mail: info@nsf.org
Website: www.nsf.org

Rain Barrels

Gardener's Supply
128 Intervale Road
Burlington, VT 05401
Tel.: (888) 833-1412
E-mail: info@gardeners.com
Website: www.gardeners.com

CHAPTER 4: COMMUNICATION

Phone Companies

Working Assets
101 Market Street, Suite 700
San Francisco, CA 94105
Tel.: toll-free (866) 225-9253
Website: www.workingassets.com

Earth Tones
Tel.: toll-free (888) EARTH-TONES
   (327-8486)
E-mail: info@earth-tones.com
Website: www.earthtones.com

Cell-Phone Recycling

Wireless Foundation
1250 Connecticut Avenue NW,
   Suite 800
Washington, DC 20036
Tel.: (202) 785-0081
Fax: (202) 467-5532
E-mail: Foundation@ctia.org
Website: www.wirelessfoundation.org

Internet Services

EcoISP
P.O. Box 1678
Boulder, CO 80306-1678
Tel.: (303) 926-0700; toll-free:
   (866) 890-4510
Fax: (303) 926-5376
E-mail: customerservice@ecoisp.com
Website: www.ecoisp.com

Recycled Paper

GreenLine Paper
631 South Pine Street
York, PA 17403
Tel.: toll-free (800) 641-1117
Fax: (717) 846-3806
Website: www.greenlinepaper.com

GreenCo
74 Cotton Mill Hill, Unit 350
Brattleboro, VT 05301
Tel.: (802) 254-7605; toll-free:
   (800) 326-2897

Treecycle Recycled Paper
P.O. Box 5086
Bozeman, MT 59717
Tel.: (406) 586-5287
E-mail: info@treecycle.com
Website: www.treecycle.com

Real Earth Environmental
P.O. Box 728
Malibu, CA 90265
Tel: (310) 457-6331; toll-free
   (800) 987-3326
Fax: (310) 457-6551
E-mail: info@treeco.com
Website: www.treeco.com

Ink-Refill Kits

Mr. Inkjet
125 Topeka
Waco, TX 76712
Tel.: (254) 399-9736; toll-free:
   (800) 887-1882

Fax: (254) 399-9738
E-mail: mrinkjet@misterinkjet.com
Website: www.misterinkjet.com

All-Ink
P.O. Box 50868
Provo, UT 84605-0868
Tel.: (801) 794-0123; toll-free:
    (888) 567-6511
Fax: (801) 794-0124
E-mail: customerservice@all-ink.com
Website: www.all-ink.com

Inksell
435 Isom Road, Suite 202
San Antonio, TX 78216
Tel.: (210) 798-0087; toll-free:
    (800) 255-0483
Fax: (210) 798-0094
E-mail: info@inksell.com
Website: www.inksell.com

Online News

Environmental News Network
2020 Milvia, Suite 411
Berkeley, CA 94704
Tel.: (510) 644-3661; toll-free:
    (888) 311-3661
Fax: (208) 475-7986
E-mail: customerservice@enn.com
Website: www.enn.com

Grist Magazine
811 First Avenue, Suite 466
Seattle, WA 98104
Tel.: (206) 876-2000
Fax: (253) 423-6487
E-mail: grist@gristmagazine.com
Website: www.gristmagazine.com

Sci-Tech Daily
Website: www.scitechdaily.com

Lycos Environmental News Service
Tel.: toll-free (800) 632-9528
E-mail: news@ens-news.com
Website: www.ens-news.com

TV Reduction

TV Turnoff Network
1601 Connecticut Avenue NW,
    Suite 303
Washington, DC 20009
Tel.: (202) 518-5556
Fax: (202) 518-5560
Website: www.tvturnoff.org

Used Books

Half.com
Website: www.half.com

Bookfinder
Website: www.bookfinder.com

Videotape Recycling

Carpel Video
429 East Patrick Street
Frederick, MD 21701
Tel.: toll-free (800) 238-4300
Website: www.carpelvideo.com

ECOMedia
Tel.: toll-free (800) 359-4601
Website: www.ecomedia.net

CHAPTER 5: MONEY, CREDIT, AND INVESTING

Credit Cards

Working Assets
101 Market Street, Suite 700
San Francisco, CA 94105
Website: www.workingassets.com/
    creditcard

Alternatives Federal Credit Union
301 West State Street
Ithaca, NY 14850
Tel.: (607) 273-4611; toll-free:
    (877) 273-AFCU
Fax: (607) 277-6391
E-mail: afcu@alternatives.org
Website: www.alternatives.org/
    visacard.html

First Savings of New Hampshire
    "Card for Kids"
1 Center Street
Exeter, NH 03833
Tel.: (603) 772-7730
Website: www.chittenden.com/
    newfsnh/per-srb.html

First USA Bank, N.A.
P.O. Box 8650
Wilmington, DE 19899-8650
Website: www.firstusa.com

The Giving Card
513 East First Street, Suite 200
Tustin, CA 92780
Tel.: (714) 505-6505
Fax: (714) 505-6502
E-mail: info@thegivingcard.com
Website: www.thegivingcard.com

Credit Unions

Self-Help Credit Union
Website: www.self-help.org

National Credit Union Administration
Website: www.ncua.gov

Credit Union National Association
5710 Mineral Point Road
Madison, WI 53705-4454
Website: www.cuna.org

National Federation of Community
    Development Credit Unions
120 Wall Street, 10th Floor
New York, NY 10005
Tel.: (212) 809-1850
Fax: (212) 809-3274
E-mail: email@natfed.org
Website: www.natfed.org

Community Banks

Boston's Wainwright Bank
63 Franklin Street
Boston, MA 02110
Tel.: (617) 478-4000; toll-free:
    (888) 428-BANK
Website: www.wainwrightbank.com

Chicago's Shore Bank
7054 South Jeffery Boulevard
Chicago, IL 60649
Tel.: toll-free (800) 669-7725
Website: www.sbk.com

Independent Community Bankers of
    America
1 Thomas Circle NW, Suite 400
Washington, DC 20003
Tel.: (202) 659-8111
E-mail: info@icba.org
Website: www.icba.org

Coalition of Community Develop-
    ment Financial Institutions
Public Ledger Building, Suite 572
620 Chestnut Street
Philadelphia, PA 19106
Tel.: (215) 923-5363 ext. 248
Website: www.cdfi.org

Social-Investing Sites

Social Funds
SRI World Group, Inc.
74 Cotton Mill Hill, Suite A-255
Brattleboro, VT 05301
Tel.: (802) 251-0500
Fax: (802) 251-0555
Website: www.socialfunds.com

Social Investment Forum
1612 K Street NW, Suite 650
Washington, DC 20006
Tel.: (202) 872-5319
Fax: (202) 822-8471
E-mail: info@socialinvest.org
Website: www.socialinvest.org

KLD Research & Analytics
Russia Wharf
530 Atlantic Avenue, 7th Floor
Boston, MA 02210
Tel.: (617) 426-5270
Fax: (617) 426-5299
Website: www.kld.com

CorpWatch
P.O. Box 29344
San Francisco, CA 94129
Tel.: (415) 561-6568
Fax: (415) 561-6493
E-mail: corpwatch@corpwatch.org
Website: www.corpwatch.org

SRI News
SRI World Group
74 Cotton Mill Hill, Suite A-255
Brattleboro, VT 05301
Tel.: (802) 251-0500
Fax: (802) 251-0555
Website: www.srinews.com

Green Money Journal
P.O. Box 67
Santa Fe, NM 87504
Tel.: (505) 988-7423
E-mail: info@greenmoneyjournal.com
Website: www.greenmoney.com

Shareholder Action Network
A Project of the Social Investment
    Forum
1612 K Street NW, Suite 650
Washington, DC 20006
Tel.: (202) 872-5313
Fax: (202) 331-8166
E-mail: san@socialinvest.org
Website: www.shareholderaction.org

Good Money
Attn: Peter Lowry
370A Granite Road
Ossipee, NH 03864
Tel.: (617) 552-3346
Website: www.goodmoney.com

Discount Brokers

Ameritrade
P.O. Box 2760
Omaha, NE 68103-2760
Tel.: toll-free (800) 454-9272
Fax: (816) 243-3769
Website: www.ameritrade.com

Datek
Attn: New Accounts Dept.
P.O. Box 2300
Jersey City, NJ 07303-2300
Tel.: toll-free (800) U2-Datek
   (823-2835)
Website: www.datek.com

Brown & Co.
Dreyfus Brokerage Services
6500 Wilshire Boulevard, 9th Floor
Los Angeles, CA 90048
Tel.: toll-free (800) 416-7113
Website: www.brownco3.com

Harris Direct
P.O. Box 2062
Jersey City, NJ 07303-9662
Tel.: toll-free (800) 825-5723
Website: www.harrisdirect.com

T D Waterhouse
P.O. Box 2630
Jersey City, NJ 07303-2630
Or:
T D Waterhouse
P.O. Box 919091
San Diego, CA 92191-9091
Tel.: toll-free (800) 934-4448
Website: www.tdwaterhouse.com

FOLIO*fn*
Customer Service Department
FOLIO*fn* Investments, Inc.
P.O. Box 3068
Merrifield, VA 22116-3068
Tel.: toll-free (888) 973-7890
Website: www.foliofn.com

Sharebuilder
Netstock Corporation
1000 124th Avenue NE
Bellevue, WA 98005
Tel.: (425) 451-4440; toll-free:
   (866) SHRBLDR (747-2537)
Fax: (425) 451-4449
Website: www.sharebuilder.com

Mutual Funds

Domini Social Investments
P.O. Box 60494
King of Prussia, PA 19406-0494
Tel.: toll-free (800) 582-6757
Website: www.domini.com

Calvert
4550 Montgomery Avenue
Bethesda, MD 20814
Tel.: toll-free (800) 368-2748
E-mail: customerservice@calvert.com
Website: www.calvertgroup.com

Green Century
29 Temple Place
Boston, MA 02111
Tel.: toll-free (800) 93-GREEN
E-mail: info@greencentury.com
Website: www.greencentury.com

MMA Praxis
1110 North Main Street

P.O. Box 483
Goshen, IN 46527
Tel.: (574) 533-9511; toll-free
    (800) 348-7468
Fax: (574) 533-5264
E-mail: memberinfo@mma-online.org
Website: www.mmapraxis.com

New Alternatives
150 Broadhollow Road
Melville, NY 11747
Tel.: toll-free (800) 423-8383
E-mail: newalternativesfund@
    compuserve.com
Website: www.newalternativesfund
    .com

Parnassus
1 Market, Steuart Tower #1600
San Francisco, CA 94105
Tel.: toll-free (800) 999-3505

Fax: (415) 778-0228
Website: www.parnassus.com

Pax World
P.O. Box 8930
Wilmington, DE 19899-8930
Tel.: toll-free (800) 767-1729
Website: www.paxfund.com

Portfolio 21
721 Ninth Avenue NW, Suite 250
Portland, OR 97209
Tel.: toll-free (877) 351-4115, ext. 21
E-mail: welcome@portfolio21.com
Website: www.portfolio21.com

Walden Asset Management
40 Court Street
Boston, MA 02108
Tel.: (617) 726-7250
Fax: (617) 227-2690
Website: www.waldenassetmgmt.com

CHAPTER 6: SHOPPING

Research

Responsible Shopper
Website: www.responsibleshopper.org

Children's Health Environmental
    Coalition
Website: www.checnet.org

General Shopping Sites

Coop America
1612 K Street NW, Suite 600
Washington, DC 20006
Tel.: (202) 872-5307; toll-free:
    (800) 58-GREEN

Fax: (202) 331-8166
Website: www.coopamerica.org

Ecomall
Website: www.ecomall.com

Green Marketplace
5801 Beacon Street, Suite #2
Pittsburgh, PA 15217
Tel.: (412) 420-6400; toll-free:
    (888) 59-EARTH
Fax: (412) 420-6404
E-mail: support@greenmarketplace
    .com
Website: www.greenmarketplace.com

Lehman's Non-Electric Catalog
P.O. Box 41
Kidron, OH 44636
Tel.: toll-free 877-GET LEHMANS
    (438-5346)
Fax: (330) 857-5785
E-mail: info@lehmans.com
Website: www.lehmans.com

Gaiam Real Goods
360 Interlocken Boulevard, Suite 300
Broomfield, CO 80021-3440
Tel.: toll-free (800) 762-7325
Website: www.realgoods.com

Shop for Change
Website: www.shopforchange.org

Clothing

Maggie's Organics
1955 Pauline Boulevard, Suite 100A
Ann Arbor, MI 48103
Tel.: toll-free (800) 609-8593
E-mail: maggies@organicclothes.com
Website: www.organicclothes.com

Fisher Henney Naturals
P.O. Box 1560
Alameda, CA 94501
Tel.: toll-free (800) 3 HENNEY
Fax: (510) 521-1637
Website: www.fhnaturals.com

Patagonia
Patagonia Mail Order
8550 White Fir Street
P.O. Box 32050
Reno, NV 89523-2050
Tel.: toll-free (800) 638-6464
Website: www.patagonia.com

Ecodragon
P.O. Box 425
Portland, ME 04112
Tel.: (207) 775-6900; toll-free:
    (888) 882-HEMP
Fax: (207) 775-6999
E-mail: info@ecodragon.com
Website: www.ecodragon.com

Decent Exposures
12554 Lake City Way NE
Seattle, WA 98125
Tel.: (206) 364-4540; toll-free:
    (800) 524-4949
Website: www.decentexposures.com

Books, Toys, and Games for Children

Chinaberry Books
2780 Via Orange Way, Suite B
Spring Valley, CA 91978
Tel.: toll-free (800) 776-2242
Fax: (619) 670-5203
Website: www.chinaberry.com

Family Pastimes
R.R. 4
Perth, Ontario
Canada K7H 3C6
Tel.: (613) 267-4819
E-mail: fp@superaje.com
Website: www.familypastimes.com

Hedgehog Farms
Tel.: (203) 730-0673
E-mail: Nancy@hedgehogfarms.com
Website: www.hedgehogfarms.com

Magic Cabin Dolls
P.O. Box 1049

Madison, VA 22727-1049
Tel.: toll-free (888) 623-3655
Website: www.magiccabindolls.com

Nova Natural
817 Chestnut Ridge Road
Chestnut Ridge, NY 10977
Tel.: (877) 668-2111
E-mail: ted@novanatural.com
Website: www.novanatural.com

Paper, Scissors, Stone
P.O. Box 428
Viroqua, WI 54665
Tel.: toll-free (888) 644-5843
Fax: (608) 637-6158
Website: www.waldorfsupplies.com

Rosie Hippo's Toys
P.O. Box 2068
Port Townsend, WA 98368
Tel.: toll-free (800) 385-2620
Fax: (360) 385-1090
E-mail: custserv@rosiehippo.com
Website: www.rosiehippo.com

Back to Basics Toys
One Memory Lane
Ridgely, MD 21685-8783
Tel.: (800) 356-5360

Gifts

Fair Trade Federation
1612 K Street NW, Suite 600
Washington, DC 20006
Tel.: (202) 872-5329
E-mail: info@fairtradefederation.org
Website: www.fairtradefederation.com

Family Farms Direct
Tel.: toll-free (888) 722-8359
E-mail: Info@FamilyFarmsDirect.com
Website: www.familyfarms-direct.com

Frontier Herbs
P.O. Box 299
3021 Seventy-eighth Street
Norway, IA 52318
Tel.: toll-free (800) 669-3275
Fax: (800) 717-4372
E-mail:
  customercare@frontierherb.com
Website: www.frontierherb.com

Sales Exchange for Refugee Rehabilita-
  tion Vocation (SERRV)
122 State Street, Suite 310
Madison, WI 53701
Tel.: toll-free (800) 422-5915
E-mail: orders@serrv.org
Website: www.serrv.org

Paints, Finishes, Etc.

AFM
Tel.: toll-free (800) 239-0321
E-mail: afm@afmsafecoat.com
Website: www.afmsafecoat.com

Bioshield
Eco Design Co.
1330 Rufina Circle
Santa Fe, NM 87507
Tel.: toll-free (800) 621-2591
Fax: (505) 438-3448
Website: www.bioshieldpaint.com

Building Supplies

Building for Health
P.O. Box 113
Carbondale, CO 81623
Tel.: toll-free (800) 292-4838
Fax: (970) 963-3318
E-mail: crose@sopris.net
Website: www.buildingforhealth.com

Environmental Construction
    Outfitters
901 East 134th Street
Bronx, NY 10454
Tel.: toll-free (800) 238-5008
Website: www.environproducts.com

Environmental Home Center
1724 Fourth Avenue S
Seattle, WA 98134
Tel.: (206) 682-7332; toll-free:
    (800) 281-9785
Fax: (206) 682-8275
E-mail: customerservice@
    environmentalhomecenter.com
Website: www.environmental
    homecenter.com

Lumber

Certified Forests Products Council
721 Ninth Avenue NW, Suite 300
Portland, OR 97209
Tel.: (503) 224-2205
Fax: (503) 224-2216
E-mail: info@certifiedwood.org
Website: www.certifiedwood.org

Scientific Certification Systems
1939 Harrison Street, Suite 400
Oakland, CA 94612

Tel.: (510) 832-1415
Fax: (510) 832-0359
Website: www.scs1.com/forestry.shtml

SmartWood
Goodwin-Baker Building
65 Millet Street, Suite 201
Richmond, VT 05477
Tel.: (802) 434-5491
Fax: (802) 434-3116
E-mail: info@smartwood.org
Website: www.smartwood.org

Treated Wood
Chemical Specialties, Inc.
1 Woodlawn Green, Suite 250
200 East Woodlawn Road
Charlotte, NC 28217
Tel.: toll-free (800) 421-8661
Fax: (704) 527-8232
Website: www.treatedwood.com

Outdoor Grilling

Peoples Woods
75 Mill Street
Cumberland, RI 02864
Tel.: toll-free (800) 729-5800
Fax: (401) 725-0006
Website: www.peopleswoods.com

Wicked Good Charcoal
Laralee Distributors
200 Elm Street
West Newfield, ME 04095
E-mail: info@wickedgoodcharcoal
    .com
Website: www.wickedgoodcharcoal
    .com

Bedding and Mattresses

Coyuchi
P.O. Box 845
Point Reyes Station, CA 94956
Tel.: (415) 663-8077; toll-free:
    (888) 418-8847
Fax: (415) 663-8104
E-mail: info@coyuchiorganic.com
Website: www.coyuchiorganic.com

Earth Sake
1425 Fourth Street
Berkeley, CA 94710
Tel.: toll-free (800) 414-8074
Fax: (510) 848-5051
E-mail: info@earthsake.com
Website: www.earthsake.com

EcoChoices
EcoPlanet-EcoChoices
P.O. Box 1491
Glendora, CA 91740
Fax: (702) 543-7003
E-mail: service@ecochoices.com
Website: www.ecochoices.com

Heart of Vermont
P.O. Box 612
131 South Main Street
Barre, VT 05641
Tel.: (802) 476-3098; toll-free:
    (800) 639-4123
Fax: (802) 479-5395
E-mail: hov@drbs.com
Website: www.heartofvermont.com

Natural Emporium
16 Lake Street
Arlington, MA 02474
Tel.: toll-free (866) 260-9675
E-mail: info@naturalemporium.com
Website: www.naturalemporium.com

Natural Home Products
P.O. Box 1677
Sebastopol, CA 95473
Tel.: (707) 824-0914
Fax: (800) 329-9398
E-mail: info@naturalhomeproducts
    .com
Website: www.naturalhomeproducts
    .com

Health and Beauty Aids

Aubrey Organics
4419 North Manhattan Avenue
Tampa, FL 33614
Tel.: toll free (800) 282-7394
Fax: (813) 876-8166
Website: www.aubrey-organics.com

Avalon
E-mail: info@avalonnaturalproducts
    .com
Website: www.avalonnaturalproducts
    .com

Aveda
Tel.: toll-free (866) 823-1425
Website: www.aveda.com

Burt's Bees
P.O. Box 13489
Durham, NC 27709
Tel.: (919) 998-5200; toll-free:
    (800) 849-7112
Fax: (919) 998-5201; toll-free:
    (800) 429-7487
Website: www.burtsbees.com

Dr. Bronner's Magic Soaps
P.O. Box 28
Escondido, CA 92033
Tel.: (760) 743-2211
Fax: (760) 745-6675
E-mail: allone@drbronner.com
Website: www.drbronner.com

Dr. Hauschka
59 North Street
Hatfield, MA 01038
Tel.: toll-free (800) 247-9907
Fax: (413) 247-0680
E-mail: holistic-skincare@
    drhauschka.com
Website: www.drhauschka.com

Essential Oils (EO)
15E Koch Road
Corte Madera, CA 94925
Tel.: (415) 945-1900; toll-free:
    (800) 570-3775
Fax: (415) 945-1910
E-mail: info@eoproducts.com
Website: www.eoproducts.com

Stila Cosmetics
Tel.: toll-free (877) 565-1299
Website: www.stilacosmetics.com

The Body Shop
Tel.: toll-free (800) BODYSHOP
    (263-9746)
E-mail: usa.info@the-body-shop.com
Website: www.thebodyshop.com

Tom's of Maine
P.O. Box 710
Kennebunk, ME 04043
Tel.: toll-free (800) FOR-TOMS
    (367-8667)

Fax: (207) 985-5656
E-mail: info@tomsofmaine.com
Website: www.toms-of-maine.com

Uncle Harry's
PMB 235
704 228th Avenue NE
Redmond, WA 98053
Tel.: (425) 643-4664
Website: www.uncleharrys.com

Weleda
175 North Route 9W
Congers, NY 10920
Tel.: toll-free (800) 241-1030
E-mail: info@weleda.com
Website: www.usa.weleda.com

Feminine-Hygiene Products

Many Moons
Tel.: toll-free (800) 916-4444
E-mail: manymoons@pacificcoast.net
Website: pacificcoast.net/
    ~manymoons/index.html

Glad Rags
P.O. Box 12648
Portland, OR 97212
Tel.: (503) 282-0436; toll-free:
    (800) 799-4523
Fax: (503) 284-9883
E-mail: orders@gladrags.com
Website: www.gladrags.com

NatraCare
Tel.: (303) 617-3476
Fax: (303) 617-3495
E-mail: natrasalesmgr@indra.com
Website: www.natracare.com

Toothbrushes

Recycline
236 Holland Street
Somerville, MA 02144
Tel.: (617) 776-8401; toll-free:
    (888) 354-7296
Fax: (617) 776-8403
E-mail: info@recycline.com
Website: www.recycline.com

Baby Care

EcoBaby
332 Coogan Way
El Cajon, CA 92020
Tel.: toll-free (888) ECOBABY
    (326-2229)
Fax: (619) 562-0199
E-mail: dottie@ecobaby.com
Website: www.ecobaby.com

CHAPTER 7: PET CARE

Earth-Friendly Pet Supplies

Earth Animal
606 Post Road East
Westport, CT 06880
Tel.: toll-free (800) 622-0260
Fax: (203) 227-8094
E-mail: ea-info@earthanimal.com
Website: www.earthanimal.com

Pet Food

Cornucopia Express
229 Wall Street
Huntington, NY 11743
Tel.: toll-free (800) PET-8280
Fax: (631) 424-3513
E-mail: cornucopex@aol.com
Website: www.cornucopiaexpress.com

Dr. Harvey's
81 First Avenue
Atlantic Highlands, NJ 07716
Tel.: (732) 291-8600; toll-free:
    (866) DOCH123 (362-4123)
Fax: (732) 291-7989
E-mail: info@drharveys.com
Website: www.drharveys.com

Natura
P.O. Box 271
Santa Clara, CA 95052-0271
Tel.: (408) 261-0770; toll-free:
    (800) 532-7261
E-mail: custserv@naturapet.com
Website: www.naturapet.com

Natural Life
412 West Saint John Street
Girard, KS 66743
Tel.: (620) 724-8012; toll-free:
    (800) 367-2391
Fax: (620) 724-8424
Website: www.nlpp.com

Nature's Recipe
Tel.: toll-free (800) 237-3856
Website: www.naturesrecipe.
    heinzpetproducts.com

Nutro Natural Choice
445 Wilson Way
City of Industry, CA 91744
Tel.: toll-free (800) 833-5330
Website: www.nutroproducts.com

Pet Guard
P.O. Box 728
Orange Park, FL 32067-0728
Tel.: toll-free (800) 874-3221
E-mail: petcare@petguard.com
Website: www.petguard.com

Precise
Tel.: toll-free (888) 4-PRECISE
Website: www.precisepet.com

Sojourner Farms Natural
1 Nineteenth Avenue S
Minneapolis, MN 55454
Tel.: (612) 343-7262; toll-free:
    (888) 867-6567
Fax: (612) 343-7263
E-mail: mail@sojos.com
Website: www.sojos.com

Solid Gold Hund-N-Flocken
315 West Bradley Avenue, Suite C
El Cajon, CA 92020
Tel.: (619) 258-1914; toll-free:
    (800) 364-4863
Fax: (619) 258-3907
E-mail: dane@solidgoldhealth.com
Website: www.solidgoldhealth.com

Wysong
1880 North Eastman Road
Midland, MI 48642-7779
Tel.: (989) 631-0009; toll-free:
    (800) 748-0188
Fax: (989) 631-8801
E-mail: wysong@tm.net
Website: www.wysong.net

Medical Resources

Alt Vet Med
Website: www.altvetmed.com

American Association of Housecall
    Veterinarians
E-mail: DVMSPAS@aol.com
Website: www.athomevet.org

American Veterinary Medical Associa-
    tion's Care for Pets
Website: www.avma.org/care4pets

Cornell University College of Veteri-
    nary Medicine website
Website: www.vet.cornell.edu/
    publicresources/animalhealth

American Animal Hospital Associa-
    tion Library
Website: www.healthypet.com

American Holistic Veterinary Medical
    Association
2218 Old Emmorton Road
Bel Air, MD 21015
Tel.: (410) 569-0795
Fax: (410) 569-2346
E-mail: office@ahvma.org
Website: www.ahvma.org

U.S. National Library of Medicine
    Pets and Pet Health
Website: www.nlm.nih.gov/
    medlineplus/petsandpethealth.html

BioNutritional Diagnostics
606 Post Road E
Westport, CT 06880
Tel.: (203) 454-4466; toll-free:
    (800) 361-2313
Fax: (203) 454-1399
E-mail: info@bnaweb.com
Website: www.bnaweb.com

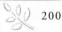

Animal Organizations

Humane Society of the United States
2100 L Street NW
Washington, DC 20037
Tel.: (202) 452-1100
Website: www.hsus.org

Animal Sanctuaries

Association of Sanctuaries (TAOS)
331 Old Blanco Road
Kendalia, TX 78027
E-mail: taos@gvtc.com
Website: www.taosanctuaries.org

CHAPTER 8: CLEANING AND HOUSEHOLD PESTS

Advocacy Groups

Children's Health Environmental
    Coalition
P.O. Box 1540
Princeton, NJ 08542
E-mail: chec@checnet.org
Website: www.checnet.org

Earth-Friendly Cleaners

Bio-Kleen
508 Harrison Street
Kalamazoo, MI 49007
Tel.: (616) 567-9400; toll-free:
    (800) 240-5536
E-mail: biokleen@net-link.net
Website: www.biokleen.com

Bon Ami
1025 West Eighth Street
Kansas City, MO 64101-1200
E-mail: info@faultless.com
Website: www.faultless.com

Citra-Solv
P.O. Box 2597
Danbury, CT 06813-2597

Tel.: (203) 778-0881; toll-free:
    (800) 343-6588
Fax: (203) 778-0911
E-mail: info@citra-solv.com
Website: www.shadowlake.com

Ecover
P.O. Box 911058
Commerce, CA 90091-1058
Tel.: toll-free (800) 449-4925
E-mail: ecover@pacbell.net
Website: www.ecover.com

Murphy's Vegetable Oil Soap
Colgate-Palmolive Co.
300 Park Avenue
New York, NY 10022-7499
Tel.: (212) 310-2000; toll-free:
    (800) 486-7627
Website: www.murphyoilsoap.com

Orange-Glo
P.O. Box 3998
Littleton, CO 80161
Tel.: toll-free (800) 781-7529
Website: www.greatcleaners.com

 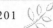

Seventh Generation
212 Battery Street, Suite A
Burlington, VT 05401-5281
Tel.: toll-free (802) 658-3773
Fax: (802) 658-1771
Website: www.seventhgen.com

General Stores

Coop America
(See chapter 6)
Website: www.coopamerica.org

EcoCities
Website: www.ecocities.net/
  shopping.htm

Homemade Cleaning Resources

Michigan State University Extension
Website: www.msue.msu.edu/msue/
  imp/mod02/01500631.html

Vermont Agency of Natural Resources
Website: www.anr.state.vt.us/
  ecosolutions/contntpg/nontoxhm.
  html

Washington Toxics Coalition
Website: www.watoxics.org/thcln.htm

Cleaning with Plants

Wolverton Environmental
514 Pine Grove Road
Picayune, MS 39466
Tel.: (601) 798-5177
Fax: (601) 798-5875
E-mail: wes.inc@datastar.net
Website:
  www.wolvertonenvironmental.com

Wet Cleaning

Professional Wet-cleaning Network
Website: www.tpwn.net

Hangers Cleaners
Cool Clean Technologies
3505 Country Road 42 W
Burnsville, MN 55306-3803
Tel.: (952) 882-5000
Website: www.hangersdrycleaners.com

Pest-Control Resources

Beyond Pesticides
National Coalition Against the Misuse
  of Pesticides
701 East Street SE #200
Washington, DC 20003
Tel.: (202) 543-5450
Fax: (202) 543-4791
E-mail: info@beyondpesticides.org
Website: www.beyondpesticides.org

Bio-Integral Resource Center
P.O. Box 7414
Berkeley, CA 94707
Tel.: (510) 524-2567
Fax: (510) 524-1758
E-mail: birc@igc.org
Website: www.birc.org

Cooper Pest Control
351 Lawrence Station Road
Lawrenceville, NJ 08648-2695
Tel.: (609) 799-1300; toll-free:
  (800) 949-2667
Fax: (609) 799-3859
E-mail: info@cooperpest.com
Website: www.cooperpest.com

CHAPTER 9: GARDENING

Magazine

Organic Gardening Magazine
33 East Minor Street
Emmaus, PA 18098
Tel.: (610) 967-5171
Website: www.organicgardening.com

Compost

Father Dom's Duck's Doo
Tel.: (262) 657-4463
Website:
    www.fatherdomsducksdoo.com

Compost Resource Page
Website: www.oldgrowth.org/compost

Worm Bins (Vermicomposting)

Gaiam Real Goods
360 Interlocken Boulevard, Suite 300
Broomfield, CO 80021-3443
Tel.: toll-free (800) 762-7325
Website: www.realgoods.com

Gardener's Supply
128 Intervale Road
Burlington, VT 05401
Tel.: (888) 833-1412
E-mail: info@gardeners.com
Website: www.gardeners.com

Seeds of Change
P.O. Box 15700
Santa Fe, NM 87592-1500
Tel.: toll-free (888) 762-7333
E-mail: soc.customer.service@
    seedsofchange.com
Website: www.seedsofchange.com

Earth-Friendly Garden Supplies

Gardens Alive
5100 Schenley Place
Lawrenceburg, IN 47025
Tel.: (812) 537-8650
Fax: (812) 537-5108
E-mail: Gardenhelp@gardensalive.com
Website: www.gardensalive.com

Planet Natural
1612 Gold Avenue
Bozeman, MT 59715
Tel.: toll-free (800) 289-6656
Fax: (406) 587-0223
E-mail: info@planetnatural.com
Website: www.planetnatural.com

Biocontrol Network
5116 Williamsburg Road
Brentwood, TN 37027
Tel.: (615) 370-4301; toll-free:
    (800) 441-2847
Fax: (615) 370-0662
E-mail: info@biconet.com
Website: www.biconet.com

Plant It Earth
33 Dorman Avenue
San Francisco, CA 94124
Tel.: (415) 970-2465
E-mail: sales@plantitearth.com
Website: www.plantitearth.com

Gardening Research

National Arboretum's U.S. Hardiness
    Zone Maps

Website: www.usna.usda.gov/
Hardzone/ushzmap.html

CRSEE: U.S. Cooperative Extension
Service Offices
Website: www.reeusda.gov/1700/
statepartners/usa.htm

EPA's Biopesticides Website
Website: www.epa.gov/pesticides/
biopesticides

USDA's Backyard Conservation advice
Website: www.nrcs.usda.gov/feature/
backyard

Native Plants

EPA's Landscaping with Native Plants
Website: www.epa.gov/greenacres

USDA's PLANTS National Database
Website: www.plants.usda.gov

Native plant societies by region:
North American Native Plant Society
P.O. Box 84, Station D
Etobicoke, Ontario
Canada M9A 4X1
Website: www.nanps.org

Online Seed Swapping

Garden Web
Website: www.gardenweb.com

Organic Gardening
33 East Minor Street
Emmaus, PA 18098
Website: www.organicgardening.com

Blossom Swap
Website: www.blossomswap.com

National Gardening
Website: www.garden.org/seedswap

Seed Companies

Burpee Seeds and Plants
300 Park Avenue
Warminster, PA 18991-0001
Tel.: toll-free (800) 333-5808
Fax: (800) 487-5530
E-mail: custserv@burpee.com
Website: www.burpee.com

Fedco Seeds
P.O. Box 520-A
Waterville, ME 04903
Fax: (207) 872-8317
Website: www.fedcoseeds.com

Johnny's Selected Seeds
184 Foss Hill Road
Albion, ME 04910
Tel.: (207) 437-4301
Fax: (800) 437-4290
E-mail:
    homegarden@johnnyseeds.com
Website: www.johnnyseeds.com

Native Seeds/SEARCH
526 North Fourth Avenue
Tucson, AZ 85705-8450
Tel.: (520) 622-5561
Fax: (520) 622-5591
E-mail: info@nativeseeds.org
Website: www.nativeseeds.org

Nichols Garden Nursery
1190 Old Salem Road NE

Albany, OR 97321-4580
Tel.: toll-free (800) 422-3985
Fax: toll-free (800) 231-5306
Website: www.nicholsgardennursery
.com

Peaceful Valley Farm Supply
P.O. Box 2209
Grass Valley, CA 95945
Tel.: (530) 272-4769; toll-free:
(888) 784-1722
Website: www.groworganic.com

Pinetree Seeds
P.O. Box 300
New Gloucester, ME 04260
Tel.: (207) 926-3400
Website: www.superseeds.com

Seeds of Change
P.O. Box 15700
Santa Fe, NM 87592-1500
Tel.: toll-free (888) 762-7333
E-mail: soc.customer.service@
seedsofchange.com
Website: www.seedsofchange.com

Seed Savers Exchange
3076 North Winn Road
Decorah, IA 52101
Tel.: (563) 382-5990
Fax: (563) 382-5872
E-mail: catalog@seedsavers.org
Website: www.seedsavers.org

Shepherd's Garden Seeds
Tel.: toll-free (800) 503-9624
Website: www.shepherdseeds.com

Stokes Seeds
P.O. Box 548

Buffalo, NY 14240-0548
Tel.: toll-free (800) 396-9238
Fax: (888) 834-3334
E-mail: stokes@stokeseeds.com
Website: www.stokeseeds.com

Territorial Seed Company
P.O. Box 158
Cottage Grove, OR 97424-0061
Tel.: (541) 942-9547
Fax: (888) 657-3131
E-mail: tertrl@territorial-seed.com
Website: www.territorial-seed.com

The Cook's Garden
P.O. Box 535
Londonderry, VT 05148
Tel.: toll-free (800) 457-9703
E-mail: info@cooksgarden.com
Website: www.cooksgarden.com

Tomato Growers Supply
P.O. Box 2237
Fort Myers, FL 33902
Tel.: toll-free (888) 478-7333
Fax: (888) 768-3476
Website: www.tomatogrowers.com

Vermont Bean Seed Company
P.O. Box 150
Vaucluse, SC 29850-0150
Tel.: toll-free (800) 349-1071
Fax: (888) 500-7333
E-mail: info@vermontbean.com
Website: www.vermontbean.com

Historic Seeds

Thomas Jefferson Center for Historic
Plants
Monticello

P.O. Box 316
Charlottesville, VA 22902
Tel.: (434) 984-9821
Website: www.twinleaf.org

Nurseries

Fieldstone Gardens
620 Quaker Lane
Vassalboro, ME 04989-9713
Tel.: (207) 923-3836
Fax: (207) 923-3836
Website: www.fieldstonegardens.com

Goodwin Creek Gardens
P.O. Box 83
Williams, OR 97544
Tel.: toll-free (800) 846-7359
Fax: (541) 846-7357
E-mail: info@goodwincreekgardens
    .com
Website: www.goodwincreekgardens
    .com

Joy Creek Nursery
20300 Watson Road NW
Scappoose, OR 97056
Tel.: (503) 543-7474
Fax: (503) 543-6933
Website: www.joycreek.com

Roslyn Nursery
211 Burrs Lane
Dix Hills, NY 11746
Tel.: (631) 643-9347
Fax: (631) 427-0894
Website: www.roslynnursery.com

Tripple Brook Farm
37 Middle Road
Southampton, MA 01073
Tel.: (413) 527-4626
Fax: (413) 527-9853
E-mail: catalog-
    request@tripplebrookfarm.com
Website: www.tripplebrookfarm.com

Well-Sweep Herb Farm
205 Mount Bethel Road
Port Murray, NJ 07865
Tel.: (908) 852-5390
Website: www.wellsweep.com

Scented Geraniums

Goodwin Creek Gardens
(See "Nurseries," above)

Geraniaceae
122 Hillcrest Avenue
Kentfield, CA 94904
Tel.: (415) 461-4168
Fax: (415) 461-7209
E-mail: geraniac@pacbell.net
Website: www.geraniaceae.com

Well-Sweep Herb Farm
(See "Nurseries," above)

Notes

CHAPTER 1: FOOD

p. 4   *ten thousand years, to the invention of agriculture:* Gary Taubes, "What If It's All Been a Big Fat Lie?" *New York Times Magazine,* 7 July 2002.

p. 5   *Few of us realize that the American . . . environment:* Frances Moore Lappé, *Diet for a Small Planet,* 20th anniversary ed. (New York: Ballantine, 1991), pp. 42–57, 61–88; Michael Pollan, *The Botany of Desire: A Plant's-Eye View of the World* (New York: Random House, 2001) pp. 183–238; and Eric Schlosser, *Fast Food Nation,* paperback ed. (New York: HarperCollins, 2001), pp. 111–166.

p. 5   *for every calorie we eat, ten calories of energy have been used:* Linda Riebel and Ken Jacobsen, *Eating to Save the Earth: Food Choices for a Healthy Planet* (Berkeley, Calif.: Celestial Arts, 2002), p. viii.

p. 5   *suicide rate among farmers and ranchers:* Schlosser, *Fast Food Nation,* p. 146.

p. 5   *In 1920, 80 percent of the consumer's dollar:* Study by Organic Farming Research Foundation

p. 5   *Since 1969, we've lost 800,000 small farms:* Ibid.

p. 6   *What the birds have taught me:* Anecdotes of pesticide effects on bird species are based on my experiences with the Santa Cruz Predatory Bird Research Group.

p. 6   *Starting in 1942 . . . wiped out:* DDT's history from Rachel Carson, *Silent Spring* (Boston: Houghton Mifflin, 1962); and Malcolm Gladwell, "The Mosquito Killer," *New Yorker,* 2 July 2001.

p. 7   *Dirty dozen:* Anne Platt McGinn, "Why Poison Ourselves? A Precautionary Approach to Synthetic Chemicals," Worldwatch Paper no. 153, Worldwatch Institute (Washington, D.C.: Dec. 2000).

p. 8   *study led by* Consumer Reports: Brian P. Baker et al., "Pesticide Residues in Conventional, IPM-Grown and Organic Foods: Insights from Three U.S. Data Sets," *Food Additives and Contaminants,* vol. 19, no. 5 (May 2002), pp. 427–446.

p. 8   *GMOs—My Biggest Concern:* My synopsis of the issues behind genetically modified organisms is based on Pollan, pp. 183–238, articles published by the GE Food Alert Campaign Center (www.gefoodalert.org), Crop Choice (www.cropchoice.com), and the Non-GMO Source (www.non-gmosource.com), and my own experiences in the industry.

p. 9   *(Bt corn) kills the insects:* Carol Kaesuk Yoon, "Reassessing Ecological Risks of Genetically Altered Plants," *New York Times,* 3 Nov. 1999; Robert C. Cowen, "New Findings Say Genetically Altered Corn Can Poison the Soil," *Christian Science Monitor,* 2 Dec. 1999; Scott Kilman, "Midwest Farmers Lose Faith They Had in Biotech Crops," *Wall Street Journal,* 19 Nov. 1999.

p. 12   *U.S. farms have lost an average of 1.7 billion tons:* Joel Makower, John Elkington, and Julia Hailes, *The Green Consumer,* rev. ed. (New York: Penguin, 1993), p. 121.

p. 14   *85 percent more likely to have birth defects:* Sandra Steingraber, "Having Faith: An Ecologist's Journey to Motherhood" (Cambridge: Perseus, 2001), pp. 113–114.

p. 19   *Twenty thousand farmworkers die:* Riebel and Jacobsen, *Eating to Save the Earth,* p. xi.

p. 19   *Organic farming is the fastest growing segment:* Ibid., p. xii.

p. 19   *Since 1900, six thousand apple varieties:* Ibid., p. xiii.

p. 21   *seventy-eight calories of fuel to create a single calorie of feedlot beef:* Lappé, *Small Planet,* p. 75.

p. 24   *12 Most Contaminated Fruits and Vegetables:* Environmental Working Group, "A Shopper's Guide to Pesticides in Produce," Chapter 2 (www.ewg.org).

p. 24   *breast cancer rates . . . prostate cancer . . . sperm counts:* Ellen Sandbeck, *Slug Bread and Beheaded Thistles: Amusing and Useful Techniques for Nontoxic Housekeeping and Gardening* (New York: Broadway Books, 2000), pp. 74, 102.

p. 24   *Childhood cancer:* Children's Health Environmental Coalition (www.checnet.org).

p. 24   *age of sexual maturity is declining:* Michael D. Lemonick, "Teens Before Their Time," *Time,* 30 Oct. 2000.

p. 24   *200 millions tons a day:* Riebel and Jacobsen, *Eating to Save the Earth,* p. x.

p. 25   *Coffee and chocolate consumed:* Fair Trade Federation; and Jean-Marie Krier, "Fair Trade in Europe 2001: Facts and Figures on the Fair Trade Sector in 18 European Countries," European Fair Trade Association (www.eftafairtrade.org). Also, from surveying articles published by the Fair Trade Foundation (www.fairtrade.org.uk), TransFair USA (www.transfairusa.org), TransFair Canada, (www.transfair.ca), and Global Exchange (www.globalexchange.org).

p. 25   *Cacao and coffee grow naturally:* Alan Davidson, *The Oxford Companion to Food* (Oxford: Oxford University Press, 1999), pp. 176–181, 201–202; and Maricel E. Presilla, *The New Taste of Chocolate* (Berkeley, Calif.: Ten Speed Press, 2001), pp. 43–55.

CHAPTER 2: TRANSPORTATION

p. 35   *Hybrid Cars Now Available:* description from Hybrid Cars (www.hybridcars.com).

p. 36   *Ford's City, muster a 50-mile range:* Ford Motor's Think Mobility Group (www.thinkmobility.com).

p. 37   *Cars and light trucks consume 40 percent. . . . The average car emits 70 tons. . . . The average U.S. car gets 27.5 miles per gallon:* Sierra Club, "The Biggest Single Step to Curbing Global Warming and Saving Oil," Sierra Club Global Warming and Energy Program.

pp. 37–38   *Streamline your car . . . keep your tires inflated properly:* Suggestions based on published materials of the U.S. Department of Energy and the Environmental Protection Agency (www.fueleconomy.gov).

p. 38   *you've saved twenty "passenger miles":* Denis Hayes, *The Official Earth Day Guide to Planet Repair* (Washington, D.C.: Island Press, 2000), pp. 68–70.

p. 38   *160-pound person burns 317 calories:* Data on calories burned during various forms of exercise vary slightly among computer calculators, and of course from person to person. We consulted the "Calories Burned" calculator presented by Health Status (www.healthstatus.com), which uses algorithms developed by the Healthier People project at Emory University's Carter Center.

CHAPTER 3: ENERGY AND WATER

p. 43   *Generating electricity . . . 100,000 deaths each year:* Center for Resource Solutions, Green-e Renewable Electricity Certification Program, "Your Health" (www.green-e.org); and "Environment: How Electricity Generation Affects Our Environment" (www.green-e.org).

p. 43   *Sulfur dioxide . . . nitrogen oxide:* U.S. Environmental Protection Agency (www.epa.gov).

p. 44   *power plants emit one ton of CO_2 per person . . . produces 25 percent of the earth's CO_2:* World Resources Institute, "The Hidden Benefits of Climate Policy: Reducing Fossil Fuel Use Saves Lives Now" (www.wri.org).

p. 44   *Radioactive waste, the dangerous debris:* Helen Caldicott, *If You Love This Planet* (New York: W. W. Norton, 1992), p. 92.

p. 45   *six billion tons worldwide at the current rate:* Ashley T. Mattoon, "Bogging Down in the Sinks," *Worldwatch* Nov./Dec. 1998.

p. 45   *earth's temperatures have risen about 1 degree Fahrenheit:* Environmental Protection Agency, "How Will Climate Change Affect the Mid-Atlantic Region?" June 2001.

p. 45   *3 to 11 degrees on average:* Intergovernmental Panel on Climate Change, "Summary for Policymakers, Climate Change 2001: Impacts, Adaptation, and Vulnerability," Report of the Working Group II of the IPCC, Feb. 2001.

p. 45   *In Alaska the average temperature . . . decimate forests:* Timothy Egan, "Alaska, No Longer So Frigid, Starts to Crack, Burn, and Sag," *New York Times,* 16 June 2002.

p. 45   *In the Alps, glaciers have shrunk:* Worldwatch Institute, "Melting of Earth's Ice Cover Reaches New High," press release, 6 March 2000 (www.worldwatch.org).

p. 45   *In Antarctica a major ice shelf:* "Icebergs Dead Ahead! Mariners Concerned About Peril of Floating Connecticut-Size Masses," CNNfyi.com, 17 May 2000.

p. 46   *A pattern of devastating floods and droughts:* Joseph D'Agnese, "Why Has Our Weather Gone Wild?" *Discover,* July 2000.

p. 46   *West Nile virus:* Ibid.

p. 46   *By September 1999 the hole over the South Pole:* United Nations Environmental Program, *Action on Ozone,* 2000 report.

p. 46   *twelve million Americans will contract skin cancer:* Greenpeace, "Our Radiant Planet: The Dangers of UV-B Radiation for Human Health and the Global Biosphere; Our Endangered Skin" (www.greenpeace.org/~ozone/radiant/).

p. 47   *the earth's remaining oil reserves:* American Petroleum Institute, "Oil Supplies: Are We Really Running Out of Oil?" (www.api.org/consumer/runningout.htm); Randy Udall and Steve Andrews, "When Will the Joyride End?" *Home Power,* newsletter, no. 81 (Feb./March 2001), Community Office for Resource Efficiency; and World Resources Institute, "World Resources 1996–97: A Guide to the Global Environment" (www.wri.org).

p. 47   *Proven natural-gas reserves . . . coal another two hundred:* Energy Information Administration, "Coal Quick Facts" and "Inventory of Electric Utility Power Plants in the United States 1999," (www.eia.doe.gov).

p. 47   *In one day the sun bombards the earth:* U.S. National Renewable Energy Laboratory, "Solar Energy: Tapping into Earth's Largest Energy Source," Dec. 1998 (www.nrel.gov/lab/pao/solar_energy.html).

p. 48   *sun supplies less than 1 percent:* U.S. Energy Information Administration, "Inventory of Electric Utility Power Plants in the United States 1999."

p. 48   *homes can be designed more efficiently:* Caldicott, *If You Love,* p. 33.

p. 48   *Living off the Grid:* Sage Mountain Center, Butte, Montana.

p. 49   *Wind is now the fastest-growing form of energy . . . close behind:* Joe Dolce, "Harvesting the Wind," *Organic Style,* March/April 2002.

p. 49   *Ireland is building:* Bijal P. Trivedi, "Ireland to Build World's Largest Wind Farm," *National Geographic Today,* 15 Jan. 2002.

p. 49   *In the United States, a New England firm:* Karen Lee Ziner, "Offshore Harvest of Wind Is Proposed for Cape Cod," *New York Times,* 3 Nov. 1999.

p. 50   *average American family flushes:* Buzz Buzzelli et al., *How to Get Water Smart: Products and Practices for Saving Water in the Nineties* (Santa Barbara, Calif.: Terra Firma, 1991), pp. 13–26.

p. 50   *Each day the average American uses:* U.S. Geologic Survey, "Water Science for Schools: Water Q & A: Water Use at Home"; U.S. Environmental Protection Agency Office of Water, "Water Facts," Dec. 1999.

p. 50   *One billion people ... three million people:* World Bank Group, "Water Help," 2001 (www.worldbank.org).

p. 51   *Switch your electricity supply to "green power":* U.S. Department of Energy, Green Power Network.

p. 53   *Compact fluorescents ... 75 percent less energy:* U.S. Environmental Protection Agency/Department of Energy Energy Star Program (www.energystar.gov).

p. 53   *total lifetime savings of forty-five dollars per bulb:* Retail claims of Philips Earthlight assume three to four hours of daily use, seven days a week. New Philips Marathon bulbs boast a six- to seven-thousand-hour life span.

p. 53   *halogen lamps have been implicated:* Lawrence Berkeley National Laboratory, "LBNL Develops Energy-Efficient CFL Torchiere," Lighting Systems Research Group (www.eetd.lbl.gov).

p. 54   *Help your heater do its best:* Alex Wilson, Jennifer Thorne, and John Morrill, *Consumer Guide to Home Energy Saving,* 7th ed. (Washington, D.C.: American Council for an Energy-Efficient Economy, 1999), pp. 41–89.

p. 55   *electrostatic air filter ... clean them regularly:* Retailer claim of ERAMCO, Inc., Dust Free, Royse City, Tex. (www.dustfree.com).

p. 55   *program your automatic thermostat:* U.S. Department of Energy, Office of Energy Efficiency and Renewable Energy Clearinghouse (EREC), "Automatic and Programmable Thermostats" fact sheet, March 1997.

p. 56   *Refrigerator wisdom:* Wilson, Thorne, and Morrill, *Home Energy Saving,* pp. 137–144; U.S. Department of Energy Energy Star Program; Department of Energy, "About DOE's Appliance Standards Program," and "Why Buy Energy Efficient Appliances?"

p. 56   *Cooking tips:* Wilson, Thorne, and Morrill, *Home Energy Saving,* pp. 145–151; U.S. Department of Energy, "Why Buy"; and U.S. Department of Energy Energy Star Program.

p. 57   *Clothes dryers gobble up 10 percent:* Caldicott, *If You Love,* p. 35.

p. 58   *Seal your envelope:* U.S. Department of Energy, "Energy-Efficient Windows," Office of Energy Efficiency and Renewable Energy Clearinghouse, fact sheet, Oct. 1994.

p. 60   *Plant "energy trees":* "Plant a Tree, Cut Your Energy Bill," *Organic Gardening,* March/April 2002.

p. 63   *foam insulation in U.S. fridges:* Greenpeace, "Greenfreeze: A Revolution in Domestic Refrigeration," Greenpeace Ozone Project.

p. 63   *HFCs ... the most potent greenhouse gases:* U.S. Environmental Protection Agency Ozone Depletion Glossary.

p. 63   *new gases not due to be phased out until 2030:* U.S. Environmental Protection Agency Ozone Depletion Office, "HCFC Phaseout Schedule."

p. 63   *refrigerants continue to be traded on international black markets:* Don Robertson, "Illegal Imports of Banned CFCs on the Rise," South Africa *Sunday Times,* 5 July 1998.

p. 66   *The deal with drinking water:* Colin Ingram, *The Drinking Water Book: A Complete Guide to Safe Drinking Water* (Berkeley, Calif.: Ten Speed Press, 1991); and Natural Resources Defense Council, "Bottled Water: Pure Drink or Pure Hype?" March 1999 (www.nrdc.org).

p. 67   *Federal standards now require new showerheads:* Scott Chaplin, "Water Efficiency: The Next Generation," Rocky Mountain Institute, draft 5-93 (1998) (www.rmi.org).

p. 67   *A plastic toilet dam inserted into an old tank:* Rutgers Cooperative Extension, "Water Conservation for Homes, Institutions, and Businesses."

p. 67   *Older toilets waste as much as 7 gallons per flush:* Chaplin, "Water Efficiency"; and Buzzelli, "Water Smart," pp. 13–26.

CHAPTER 4: COMMUNICATION

p. 77   *One ton (forty cartons) . . . saves 7.2 trees:* Conservatree, "Trees into Paper: How Much Paper Can Be Made from a Tree?" (www.conservatree.com).

p. 77   *One ton of 50 percent postconsumer . . . saves 12 trees:* Ibid.

p. 79   *Mounting Tide of Mobiles:* Peter Nulty, *Strong Signals,* newsletter, Strong Funds, 15 May 2002 and 24 May 2002.

p. 80   *One ream—five hundred sheets—uses up 6 percent of a tree:* Conservatree, "Trees into Paper."

p. 81   *40 percent of all the solid waste generated:* Recycled Paper Coalition (www.papercoalition.org).

p. 82   *Dioxins have been shown to be carcinogenic:* Anne Platt McGinn, "Why Poison Ourselves? A Precautionary Approach to Synthetic Chemicals," Worldwatch Paper no. 153, Worldwatch Institute, Washington, D.C., Nov. 2000, p. 18–28; Helen Caldicott, *If You Love This Planet* (New York: W. W. Norton, 1992), pp. 56–59; and Sandra Steingraber, *Having Faith: An Ecologist's Journey to Motherhood* (Cambridge: Perseus, 2001), pp. 299–300.

p. 83   *Alternative fibers such as hemp, flax, and kenaf:* Hemp Industries Association (www.thehia.org); Flax Council of Canada (www.flax council.ca); and the American Kenaf Society (www.kenaf society.org).

p. 84   *American kids watch twenty-one hours of TV:* Eric Schlosser, *Fast Food Nation,* paperback ed. (New York: HarperCollins, 2001), p. 46.

CHAPTER 5: MONEY, CREDIT, AND INVESTING

p. 87   *Sixty-one percent of Americans invest:* James Glassman, "Small Investors Show Grace Under Pressure," *American Enterprise Online,* Jan./Feb. 2002.

p. 87   *Fifty million households own mutual funds . . . $27 trillion:* Richard W. Fisher, "Warren Buffett and the American Dream," *Globalist,* 30 May 2001.

p. 88   *Bad corporate citizens:* Brian Bremner, "No Cheer in Japan Over America's Woes," *Business Week,* 11 July 2002; Amy Borrus et al., "What Corporate Cleanup?" *Business Week,* 7 June 2002; and Mike McNamee, "The SEC Isn't Answering Investors' Prayers," *Business Week,* 7 June 2002.

p. 90   *top ten holdings:* KLD, Boston (www.kld.com).

p. 94   *Almost one out of every eight dollars:* Social Investment Forum, *2001 Trends Report.*

p. 94   *More than $900 billion in assets:* Ibid.

p. 96   *In its first ten years, the Domini 400 Social Index:* KLD, Boston.

CHAPTER 6: SHOPPING

p. 107   *Great Wall became dwarfed by the Fresh Kills Landfill:* "A Brief History of Recycling," *Christian Science Monitor,* 17 April 2002.

p. 107   *This "peak" is the highest geographic feature:* William Rathje and Cullen Murphy, *Rubbish! The Archaeology of Garbage* (Tucson: University of Arizona Press, 2001), pp. 4–5.

p. 107   *thirty-year-old phone books:* Rathje and Murphy, *Rubbish!* These are just the beginning of the finds unearthed by archaeologist William Rathje and his fellow "garbologists." It was Rathje's work that dispelled the myth that garbage biodegrades in landfills. His research also shows that paper, not plastic, makes up the greater bulk of American trash heaps.

p. 107   *Cotton is grown on 3 to 5 percent . . . 25 percent of the world's pesticide each year:* Cally Law, "The Poisoned Legacy of the Cotton T-Shirt," London *Times,* 26 April 2000; and Organic Trade Association.

p. 108   *Bená Burda was searching:* Story of the Maquilador Mujeres, the Nicaraguan sewing cooperative, based on interviews with Bená Burda and Jody Milano, and unreleased video footage.

p. 109   *chemicals called phthalates:* Children's Health Environmental Coalition (www.checnet.org/healthehouse); and U.S. Environmental Protection Agency, "The Inside Story: A Guide to Indoor Air Quality" (www.epa.gov).

p. 111   *groups have advocated limiting exposure to a number of chemicals:* Aubrey Hampton, *What's in Your Cosmetics? A Complete Consumer's Guide to Natural and Synthetic Ingredients* (Tucson: Odonian Press, 1995), pp. 6–183; and David Steinman and Samuel S. Epstein, *The Safe Shopper's Bible: A Consumer's Guide to Nontoxic Household Products, Cosmetics, and Food* (New York: Macmillan, 1995), pp. 181–291.

p. 112   *Fifty-three percent of Americans . . . but don't know how: Roper Green Gauge Report,* as cited by U.S. Department of Energy's Green Power site (www.eren.doe.gov/greenpower).

p. 114   *Bag the Bags!:* Lovekit Dhaliwal, "Bombay Gets Tough on Plastic Bags," BBC News, 14 May 2001; and other BBC News stories (unsigned) regarding plastic bags.

CHAPTER 7: PET CARE

p. 118   *the four D's: dead, diseased, disabled, or dying livestock:* Animal Protection Institute, "What's Really in Pet Food?" 1 Jan. 2002.

p. 118   *In Europe mad-cow disease:* Eric Schlosser, *Fast Food Nation,* paperback ed. (New York: HarperCollins, 2001), pp. 271–288.

p. 118   *carcasses may be sold . . . and end up in pet food:* Stephanie Simon, "Outcry Over Pets in Pet Food," *Los Angeles Times,* 6 Jan. 2002; and U.S. Food and Drug Administration, "Report on the Risk from Pentobarbital in Dog Food," FDA Center for Veterinary Medicine, 1 March 2002.

p. 118   *traces of barbiturates:* Ibid.

p. 118   *discarded restaurant grease:* Buck Wolf, "From Fast Food to Dog Food," Wolf files, ABC News.com (www.abcnews.go.com).

p. 123   *Flavor enhancers, snacks, juices, etc.:* Robert S. Goldstein and Susan J. Goldstein, "Super Foods and Healing Meals for Your Pets," *Love of Animals,* newsletter.

p. 124   *Keep air fresh. . . . Learn animal first aid:* Robert S. Goldstein and Susan J. Goldstein, "137 Astonishing Health Secrets for Your Pet," *Love of Animals,* newsletter.

p. 125   *$11 billion-a-year industry:* Animal Protection Institute, 1 Jan. 2002 (www.api4animals.org).

p. 125   *Ninety percent of vets surveyed:* Survey by the Animal Protection Institute and the Association of Veterinarians for Animal Rights (AVAR), spring 1998.

p. 125   *Cancer is the number one disease:* CVM Today, "What Is the Incidence of Cancer in Our Pets?" and "Cancer in Animals," both Texas A&M College of Veterinary Medicine, winter 2000.

p. 125   *Twenty-five percent of all animal-shelter pets are purebred:* Humane Society of the United States.

p. 125   *In seven years, a fertile cat and her offspring:* Ibid.

p. 127   *our pets comprise 80 percent:* D'Agnese, "Aerospace: Paul MacCreaty, Designer of the First Human-Powered Aircraft," *Discover,* July 2002.

p. 127   *eight to ten million animals:* Humane Society of the United States.

CHAPTER 8: CLEANING AND HOUSEHOLD PESTS

p. 136   *What About Dry Cleaning?:* U.S. Environmental Protection Agency, "Chemicals in the Environment: What Is Perchloroethylene, How Is It Used, and How Might I Be Exposed?" 11 Oct. 2001; Greenpeace, "Dry Cleaning Chemical Linked to Hundreds of Deaths, Warrants EPA Listing as Carcinogen," press release 11 July 2001; and Children's Health Environmental Coalition's Healthe-House site (www.checnet.org).

p. 136   *The EPA says the air in the average home:* Margot Higgins, "Earth Day Advice: Be Smart with Spring Cleaning," Environmental News Network, 17 April 2001.

p. 137   *seventy to eighty thousand chemicals:* "People Harmed by Toxic

Chemicals v. Chemical Companies: Thousands of Deaths Yearly from Toxic Chemicals," a summary of class-action suits dating to 2001, Class Action America (www.classactionamerica.com); and U.S. Environmental Protection Agency's Chemical Testing and Information Home Page, Office of Pollution Prevention and Toxics.

p. 137 *"A recent EPA study":* "Chemical Hazard Data Availability Study: High Production Volume (HPV) Chemicals and SIDS Testing," U.S. Environmental Protection Agency Office of Pollution Prevention and Toxics, April 1998.

p. 138 *Are kids at risk?* "Did You Know? Interesting Facts About Children's Environmental Health," a summary of facts from leading reports, Children's Environmental Health Coalition (www.checnet.org).

p. 139 *Plants That Clean Air:* B. C. Wolverton, *How to Grow Fresh Air: 50 Houseplants That Purify Your Home or Office* (New York: Penguin, 1997), pp. 40–58.

p. 140 *Reading Labels:* "How Toxic Is Toxic?", public fact sheet by the Merced County Association of Governments, Merced, Calif.; and Wilma Hammet, "Hazardous Household Products: How Do You Know if a Product Is Hazardous?" North Carolina Cooperative Extension Service, March 1996.

p. 141 *Replace conventional cleaning products with homemade cleaners:* Philip Dickey, "Safer Cleaning Products," Washington Toxics Coalition, Seattle (www.watoxics.org); U.S. Environmental Protection Agency, "Hazardous Waste: Common Cleaning Products"; Gary A. Davis and Em Turner, "Fact Sheet: Safe Substitutes at Home: Non-Toxic Household Products," Michigan State University Extension Service; and Wilma Hammet, "Cleaning Recipes for a Healthy Home," North Carolina Cooperative Extension Service, Jan. 1991.

p. 142 *The Worst Offenders:* Hammet, "Hazardous Household Products"; and Richard Alexander, "The Top 10 Hazardous Household Chemicals," *Consumer Law Page,* 1994.

CHAPTER 9: GARDENING

p. 162 *Banish pests on the cheap:* For ideas, see Ellen Sandbeck, *Slug Bread and Beheaded Thistles: Amusing and Useful Techniques for Nontoxic Housekeeping and Gardening* (New York: Broadway Books, 2000).

p. 164 *We Americans lavish more than thirty billion dollars:* Michael Pollan,

Second Nature: A Gardener's Education (New York: Laurel, 1992), p. 66.

p. 164   *Thirty percent of all water:* National Wildlife Federation, "Problems Associated with Traditional Landscaping," fact sheet.

p. 164   *Seventy million pounds of chemicals:* Ibid.

p. 164   *mowers . . . emit as much hydrocarbon:* Ibid.

p. 171   *A Child's Garden:* Mel Bartholomew, *Square Foot Gardening* (Emmaus, Penn.: Rodale, 1981), pp. 243–246; and Sherry Mitchell, *The Townhouse Gardener: Distinctive Landscapes for Small Gardens in the Mid-Atlantic Region* (McLean, Va.: EPM, 1998), pp. 64–65.

EPILOGUE: GENEROSITY

p. 178   *Since 1985, they have given:* Patagonia.

Bibliography

BOOKS

Bartholomew, Mel. *Square Foot Gardening.* Emmaus, Penn.: Rodale, 1981.

Berthold-Bond, Annie. *Clean & Green: The Complete Guide to Nontoxic and Environmentally Safe Housekeeping.* Woodstock, N.Y.: Ceres Press, 1990.

Buzzelli, Buzz, et al. *How to Get Water Smart: Products and Practices for Saving Water in the Nineties.* Santa Barbara, Calif.: Terra Firma, 1991.

Caldicott, Helen. *The New Nuclear Danger.* New York: New Press, 2002.

———. *If You Love This Planet.* New York: W. W. Norton, 1992.

Carson, Rachel. *Silent Spring.* Boston: Houghton Mifflin, 1962. (Crest Reprint, 1964).

Dacyczyn, Amy. *The Complete Tightwad Gazette: Promoting Thrift as a Viable Alternative Lifestyle.* New York: Random House, 1999.

Damrosch, Barbara. *The Garden Primer.* New York: Workman, 1998.

Davidson, Alan. *The Oxford Companion to Food.* Oxford: Oxford University Press, 1999.

Dominguez, Joe, and Vicki Robin. *Your Money or Your Life: Transforming Your Relationship with Money and Achieving Financial Independence.* New York: Penguin, 1999.

Domini, Amy. *Socially Responsible Investing: Making a Difference and Making Money.* Chicago: Dearborn Trade, 2001.

Giono, Jean. *The Man Who Planted Trees.* White River Junction, Vt.: Chelsea Green, 1985.

Goldstein, Martin. *The Nature of Animal Healing: The Definitive Holistic Medicine Guide to Caring for Your Dog and Cat.* New York: Ballantine, 2000.

Gussow, Joan Dye. *This Organic Life: Confessions of a Suburban Homesteader.* White River Junction, Vt.: Chelsea Green, 2001.

Hampton, Aubrey. *What's in Your Cosmetics? A Complete Consumer's Guide to Natural and Synthetic Ingredients.* Tucson, Ariz.: Odonian Press, 1995.

Hayes, Denis. *The Official Earth Day Guide to Planet Repair.* Washington, D.C.: Island Press, 2000.

Ingram, Colin. *The Drinking Water Book: A Complete Guide to Safe Drinking Water.* Berkeley, Calif.: Ten Speed Press, 1991.

Keats, John. *The Insolent Chariots.* Philadelphia: Lippincott, 1958.

———. *What Ever Happened to Mom's Apple Pie? The American Food Industry and How to Cope with It.* Boston: Houghton Mifflin, 1976.

Lappé, Frances Moore. *Diet for a Small Planet.* 20th anniversary ed. New York: Ballantine, 1991.

Makower, Joel, with John Elkington and Julia Hailes. *The Green Consumer.* Rev. ed. New York: Penguin USA, 1993.

Mander, Jerry. *Four Arguments for the Elimination of Television.* New York: Morrow Quill Paperbacks, 1997.

Mitchell, Henry. *The Essential Earthman.* Bloomington: Indiana University Press, 1981.

Mitchell, Sherry. *The Townhouse Gardener: Distinctive Landscapes for Small Gardens in the Mid-Atlantic Region.* McLean, Va.: EPM Publications, 1998.

Nader, Ralph. *Unsafe at Any Speed: The Designed-In Dangers of the American Automobile.* New York: Grossman, 1966.

Pollan, Michael. *Second Nature: A Gardener's Education.* New York: Laurel, 1992.

———. *The Botany of Desire: A Plant's-Eye View of the World.* New York: Random House, 2001.

Presilla, Maricel E. *The New Taste of Chocolate.* Berkeley, Calif.: Ten Speed Press, 2001.

Rathje, William, and Cullen Murphy. *Rubbish! The Archaeology of Garbage.* Tucson: University of Arizona Press, 2001.

Reich, Lee. *Weedless Gardening.* New York: Workman Publishing, 2001.

Riebel, Linda, and Ken Jacobsen. *Eating to Save the Earth: Food Choices for a Healthy Planet.* Berkeley, Calif.: Celestial Arts, 2002.

Sandbeck, Ellen. *Slug Bread and Beheaded Thistles: Amusing and Useful Techniques for Nontoxic Housekeeping and Gardening.* New York: Broadway Books, 2000.

Schlosser, Eric. *Fast Food Nation.* Paperback ed. New York: HarperCollins, 2001.

Steingraber, Sandra. *Having Faith: An Ecologist's Journey to Motherhood.* Cambridge: Perseus, 2001.

Steinman, David, and Samuel S. Epstein. *The Safe Shopper's Bible: A Consumer's Guide to Nontoxic Household Products, Cosmetics, and Food.* New York: Macmillan, 1995.

Wilson, Alex, Jennifer Thorne, and John Morrill. *Consumer Guide to Home Energy Saving.* 7th ed. Washington, D.C.: American Council for an Energy-Efficient Economy, 1999.

Wolverton, B. C. *How to Grow Fresh Air: 50 Houseplants That Purify Your Home or Office.* New York: Penguin, 1997.

MEDIA ARTICLES

BBC News. "A World Drowning in Litter." 4 March 2002.

———. "Northern Ireland Shoppers Would Bring Their Own Bags." 4 March 2002.

———. "Planet Earth's New Nemesis?" 8 May 2002.

———. "Taiwan to Ban Plastic Bags." 3 Oct. 2001.

———. "Tax on Plastic Bags Considered." 6 May 2002.

Borrus, Amy, et al. "What Corporate Cleanup?" *Business Week,* 7 June 2002 (www.businessweek.com).

Bremner, Brian. "No Cheer in Japan Over America's Woes." *Business Week,* 11 July 2002 (www.businessweek.com).

Christian Science Monitor. "A Brief History of Recycling." 17 April 2002.

CNNfyi.com. "Icebergs Dead Ahead! Mariners Concerned About Peril of Floating Connecticut-Size Masses," 17 May 2000.

Cowen, Robert C. "New Findings Say Genetically Altered Corn Can Poison the Soil." *Christian Science Monitor,* 2 Dec. 1999.

D'Agnese, Joseph. "Aerospace: Paul MacCready, Designer of the First Human-Powered Aircraft." *Discover,* July 2002.

———. "Why Has Our Weather Gone Wild?" *Discover,* July 2000.

Dhaliwal, Lovekit. "Bombay Gets Tough on Plastic Bags." BBC News, 14 May 2001.

Dolce, Joe. "Harvesting the Wind." *Organic Style,* March/April 2002.

Egan, Timothy. "Alaska, No Longer So Frigid, Starts to Crack, Burn and Sag." *New York Times,* 16 June 2002.

Fisher, Richard W. "Warren Buffett and the American Dream." *Globalist,* 30 May 2001.

Gladwell, Malcolm. "The Mosquito Killer." *New Yorker,* 2 July 2001.

Glassman, James. "Small Investors Show Grace Under Pressure." *American Enterprise Online,* Jan./Feb. 2002.

Goldstein, Robert S., and Susan J. Goldstein. "137 Astonishing Health Secrets for Your Pet." *Love of Animals,* newsletter.

———. "Super Foods and Healing Meals for Your Pets," *Love of Animals,* newsletter.

Higgins, Margot. "Earth Day Advice: Be Smart with Spring Cleaning." Environmental News Network, 17 April 2001.

Kilman, Scott. "Midwest Farmers Lose Faith They Had in Biotech Crops." *Wall Street Journal,* 19 Nov. 1999.

Law, Cally. "The Poisoned Legacy of the Cotton T-Shirt." *London Times,* 26 April 2000.

Lemonick, Michael D. "Teens Before Their Time." *Time,* 30 Oct. 2000.

Mattoon, Ashley T. "Bogging Down in the Sinks." *Worldwatch,* Nov./Dec. 1998.

McNamee, Mike. "The SEC Isn't Answering Investors' Prayers." *Business Week,* 7 June 2002 (www.businessweek.com).

Nulty, Peter. *Strong Signals.* Newsletter, Strong Funds, 15 May and 24 May 2002.

Organic Gardening. "Plant a Tree, Cut Your Energy Bill." March/April 2002.

Robertson, Don. "Illegal Imports of Banned CFCs on the Rise." (South Africa) *Sunday Times,* 5 July 1998 (www.btimes.co.za).

Simon, Stephanie. "Outcry Over Pets in Pet Food." *Los Angeles Times,* 6 Jan. 2002.

Taubes, Gary. "What If It's All Been a Big Fat Lie?" *New York Times Magazine,* 7 July, 2002.

Trivedi, Bijal P. "Ireland to Build World's Largest Wind Farm." *National Geographic Today,* 15 Jan. 2002 (www.news.nationalgeographic.com).

Wolf, Buck. "From Fast Food to Dog Food." Wolf Files, ABC News.com.

Yoon, Carol Kaesuk. "Reassessing Ecological Risks of Genetically Altered Plants." *New York Times,* 3 Nov. 1999.

Ziner, Karen Lee. "Offshore Harvest of Wind Is Proposed for Cape Cod." *New York Times,* 16 April 2002.

SCIENTIFIC PAPERS, GOVERNMENT AND NGO REPORTS

Alexander, Richard. "The Top 10 Hazardous Household Chemicals." *Consumer Law Page,* 1994.

American Petroleum Institute. "Oil Supplies: Are We Really Running Out of Oil?" (www.api.org).

Animal Protection Institute. "What's Really in Pet Food?" 1 Jan. 2002 (www.api4animals.org).

Baker, Brian P., et al. "Pesticide Residues in Conventional, IPM-Grown and Organic Foods: Insights from Three U.S. Data Sets." *Food Additives and Contaminants,* vol. 19, no. 5 (May 2002): 427–446.

Center for Alternative Technology. "Making Use of Waste Water." Tipsheet 6, 1997 (www.cat.org.uk).

Chaplin, Scott. "Water Efficiency: The Next Generation." Rocky Mountain Institute, Draft 5-93, 1998 (www.rmi.org).

Conservatree. "Trees into Paper: How Much Paper Can Be Made from a Tree?" (www.conservatree.com).

CVM Today. "Cancer in Animals." Texas A&M College of Veterinary Medicine, winter 2000 (www.cvm.tamu.edu/cvmtoday).

———. "What Is the Incidence of Cancer in Our Pets?" Texas A&M College of Veterinary Medicine, winter 2000 (www.cvm.tamu.edu/oncology).

Davis, Gary A., and Em Turner. "Fact Sheet: Safe Substitutes at Home: Non-Toxic Household Products." U.S. Environmental Protection Agency with the permission of the Tennessee Valley Authority, Regional Waste Management Department.

Dickey, Philip. "Safer Cleaning Products." Washington Toxics Coalition, Seattle (www.watoxics.org).

Dunn, Seth. "Hydrogen Futures: Toward a Sustainable Energy System." Worldwatch Paper no. 157 (Aug. 2001), Worldwatch Institute, Washington, D.C.

Environmental Working Group. "A Shopper's Guide to Pesticides in Produce." Washington, D.C. (www.ewg.org).

Fair Trade Federation. *2002 Report on Fair Trade Trends in the U.S. and Canada* (www.fairtradefederation.com).

Goodridge, Jim. "One Hundred Years of Rainfall Trends in California." Watershed Management Council (www.watershed.org).

Greenpeace. "Our Radiant Planet: The Dangers of UV-B Radiation for Human Health and the Global Biosphere; Our Endangered Skin" (www.greenpeace.org).

———. "Dry Cleaning Chemical Linked to Hundreds of Deaths, Warrants EPA Listing as Carcinogen." Press release, 11 July 2001 (www.greenpeaceusa.org).

———. "Greenfreeze: A Revolution in Domestic Refrigeration." Greenpeace Ozone Project (www.greenpeace.org).

Hammet, Wilma. "Cleaning Recipes for a Healthy Home." North Carolina Cooperative Extension Service, Jan. 1991.

———. "Hazardous Household Products: How Do You Know if a Product Is Hazardous?" North Carolina Cooperative Extension Service, March 1996.

Humane Society of the United States. Pet Overpopulation Estimates (www.hsus.org).

Intergovernmental Panel on Climate Change. "Summary for Policymakers, Climate Change 2001: Impacts, Adaptation, and Vulnerability." Report of the Working Group II of the IPCC, Feb. 2001.

Krier, Jean-Marie. "Fair Trade in Europe 2001: Facts and Figures on the Fair Trade Sector in 18 European Countries." European Fair Trade Association (www.eftafairtrade.org).

Lawrence Berkeley National Laboratory. "LBNL Develops Energy-Efficient CFL Torchiere." Lighting Systems Research Group (www.eetd.lbl.gov).

Maeder, Paul, et al. "Soil Fertility and Biodiversity in Organic Farming." *Science* 296: 1694–1697.

McGinn, Anne Platt. "Why Poison Ourselves? A Precautionary Approach to Synthetic Chemicals." Worldwatch Paper no. 153 (Nov. 2000), Worldwatch Institute, Washington, D.C.

Michigan State University Extension Service. "Homemade Cleaners: Safer Alternatives: Reducing the Risk." 4 Dec. 1998.

National Wildlife Federation. "Problems Associated with Traditional Landscaping." Fact sheet.

National Wind Coordinating Committee. "Understanding Non-Residential Demand for Green Power." Jan. 2001 Consensus Report.

Natural Resources Defense Council. "Bottled Water: Pure Drink or Pure Hype?" March 1999 (www.nrdc.org).

Organic Trade Association. "Organic Cotton Facts" (www.ota.com).

Rutgers Cooperative Extension. "Water Conservation for Homes, Institutions, and Businesses."

Sierra Club. "The Biggest Single Step to Curbing Global Warming and Saving Oil." Sierra Club Global Warming and Energy Program.

Social Investment Forum. *2001 Trends Report* (www.socialinvest.org).

U.S. Department of Energy. "About DOE's Appliance Standards Program." Office of Codes and Standards, July 2001 (www.eren.doe.gov).

———. "Energy-Efficient Windows." Fact Sheet, Office of Energy Efficiency and Renewable Energy Clearinghouse (EREC), Oct. 1994.

———. "Why Buy Energy Efficient Appliances?" Office of Codes and Standards, July 2001 (www.eren.doe.gov).

———. Energy Star Program (www.energystar.gov).

———. Green Power Network (www.eren.doe.gov/greenpower/home.shtml).

U.S. Energy Information Administration. "Natural Gas Use in American Households." Jan. 2001 (www.eia.doe.gov).

———. "Coal Quick Facts" (www.eia.doe.gov).

———. "Inventory of Electric Utility Power Plants in the United States 1999" (www.eia.doe.gov).

U.S. Environmental Protection Agency. "Chemicals in the Environment: What Is Perchloroethylene, How Is It Used, and How Might I Be Exposed?" 11 Oct. 2001 (www.epa.gov).

———. "Hazardous Waste: Common Cleaning Products."

———. "HCFC Phaseout Schedule." Ozone Depletion Office, June 1998 (www.epa.gov).

————. "How Will Climate Change Affect the Mid-Atlantic Region?" June 2001.

————. "The Inside Story: A Guide to Indoor Air Quality" (www.epa.gov).

————. "Water Facts." Office of Water, Dec. 1999.

U.S. Food and Drug Administration. "Report on the Risk from Pentobarbital in Dog Food." FDA Center for Veterinary Medicine, 1 March 2002.

U.S. Geologic Survey. "Water Science for Schools: Water Q&A: Water Use at Home."

U.S. National Renewable Energy Laboratory. "Solar Energy: Tapping into Earth's Largest Energy Source." Dec. 1998 (www.nrel.gov).

Udall, Randy, and Steve Andrews. "When Will the Joyride End?" *Home Power,* newsletter, no. 81 (Feb/March 2001), Community Office for Resource Efficiency.

United Nations Environmental Program. *Action on Ozone.* 2000 report.

World Bank Group. "Water Help." 2001 (www.worldbank.org).

World Resources Institute. "The Hidden Benefits of Climate Policy: Reducing Fossil Fuel Use Saves Lives Now" (www.wri.org).

————. "World Resources 1996–97: A Guide to the Global Environment" (www.wri.org).

Worldwatch Institute. "Melting of Earth's Ice Cover Reaches New High." Press release, 6 March 2000 (www.worldwatch.org).

Index

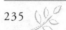

ABOUT THE AUTHORS

NELL NEWMAN launched Newman's Own Organics with business partner Peter Meehan in 1993. She is the daughter of actors Paul Newman and Joanne Woodward, from whom she received an early introduction to natural foods, environmental concerns, cooking, and fly-fishing. She attended the College of the Atlantic, graduating with a B.S. in human ecology. Before founding Newman's Own Organics, she worked at the Environmental Defense Fund, the Ventana Wilderness Sanctuary, and the Santa Cruz Predatory Bird Research Group. She lives in Santa Cruz, California.

JOSEPH D'AGNESE is a contributing editor to *Discover* magazine. His work was selected for inclusion in the 2002 edition of *The Best American Science Writing.* D'Agnese has also written for *The New York Times, This Old House, Saveur,* and *Garden Design,* among other publications. He lives in Hoboken, New Jersey.